BABY SLEEP TRAINING IN **7** DAYS

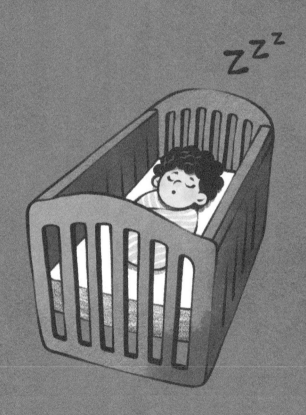

BABY SLEEP TRAINING IN 7 DAYS

The Fastest Fix for Sleepless Nights

VIOLET GIANNONE, R.N.

ALTHEA
PRESS

TO MY STRONG COFFEE
AND ITALIAN COOKIES,
MY LOYAL COMPANIONS
THROUGH THE WRITING JOURNEY.
WITHOUT YOU THIS BOOK
WOULD NOT BE POSSIBLE.

CONTENTS

Introduction ix

before the seven days

STEP 1: Survive the First Three Months. 3

STEP 2: Create a Sleep-Friendly Space. 13

STEP 3: Establish a Routine. 21

STEP 4: Choose Your Moment. 29

STEP 5: Prepare for the Seven Days. 37

during the seven days

STEP 1: Put Baby to Bed. 47

STEP 2: Check In. 51

STEP 3: Stay Strong. 57

STEP 4: Handle Night Wakings. 61

STEP 5: Repeat. 65

after the seven days

STEP 1: Manage Props 75

STEP 2: End Nighttime Snacktime 79

STEP 3: Tackle Naptime 85

STEP 4: Adapt to Changing Schedules 93

STEP 5: Conquer Setbacks 99

Epilogue 105

Resources 106

References 108

Index 110

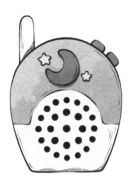

INTRODUCTION

WHEN MY DAUGHTER BRIANNA WAS BORN, I was overjoyed with the idea of being a new mom. She was perfect in every way. I couldn't wait to take on this incredible role of Mommy to my sweet baby girl. Things quickly took a turn, though, when she wouldn't sleep *at all* at night. She was literally up all night wanting to be held, rocked, or nursed back to sleep. This went on for almost a year, and in all that time, I didn't sleep more than a two-hour stretch at a time. I thought I was going insane! I was constantly anxious about bedtime, and dreaded the nighttime hours. I was exhausted, frustrated, and at my wit's end. This was not how I had imagined motherhood; I knew I had to do something.

So I started researching. That's when I learned about "sleep training," which is the process of teaching a baby to sleep well by establishing healthy sleep habits. I studied every single sleep training method, and read every sleep book and program I could get my hands on. I'm a registered nurse, so I relied on my medical knowledge about sleep cycles, disturbances, and how sleep works. I also made many phone calls to our amazing pediatrician. Finally, with all of this expertise under my belt, I began to try out some different sleep techniques. At one point I spent weeks studying and journaling Brianna's sleep habits, as if I was back in nursing school.

I tried different methods and tweaked things until—ta-da! She was sleeping through the night.

When my second baby arrived, I already had all this knowledge and knew so many tricks that getting her to sleep was a breeze. I began journaling, blogging, and sharing all of my tips on my website, VioletSleepBabySleep.com. My advice quickly attracted other parents who were struggling with the same exact problems.

Fast-forward to several years later—I now help parents all over the world reclaim their sleep and sanity! Through my website, I offer tons of tried-and-true sleep advice, as well as one-on-one consultations so parents can get a truly individualized approach to helping their baby sleep through the night.

I'm now delighted to share my knowledge and expertise with you in this seven-day guide to helping your baby sleep well, so that you can experience the same success that results in a happy and well-rested baby—not to mention a happy and well-rested you!

This book is broken down into three sections: preparing your child for sleep training, initiating the sleep training process, and ensuring good sleep habits continue into the future. The most important thing for you to know is this: Sleep training is like a puzzle. If it's missing any pieces, it will not work. You can set yourself up for success by reading and implementing all the sections of this book, so you don't miss any key puzzle pieces.

We'll start by exploring some tips on how to prepare your child for sleep training. I'll describe the seven-day plan in detail, so you'll know exactly what to do every step of the way. Then we'll dive into the process. While many babies can be sleep trained in a week, don't get discouraged if your journey is not complete after seven days—every day she will get better at it. Finally, we'll talk about what to do after the seven days, and address how to navigate some common bumps in the road going forward.

This book is aimed at the six-month- to two-year-old age group, but good sleep habits, like starting a bedtime routine and setting up a healthy sleep environment, can be implemented from day one.

One more note before we dive into the good stuff! Sleep training is not always easy. If it were, we would all have babies who slept through the night right after birth. However, sleep training a baby is incredibly rewarding, and essential for everyone's good health. Babies need sleep for proper growth and development. More visibly, we know that when a baby is tired, she is cranky and fussy, and doesn't want to practice her milestones. And let's not forget what sleep deprivation does to us as parents. Parenting a baby should be fun, not a dreadful, stressful, all-out mess! If you feel like you're hanging on by a cup of coffee, sit tight. I promise that there is no better feeling than achieving a full night's rest for both you and your baby.

before the seven days

As you wrap your head around the dream of sleeping through the night, I'm going to introduce you to the things you can do to set the stage, the timing, and even the lighting for your household's own production of *Sleeping Beauty!*

1 **survive the first three months**

2 **create a sleep-friendly space**

3 **establish a routine**

4 **choose your moment**

5 **prepare for the seven days**

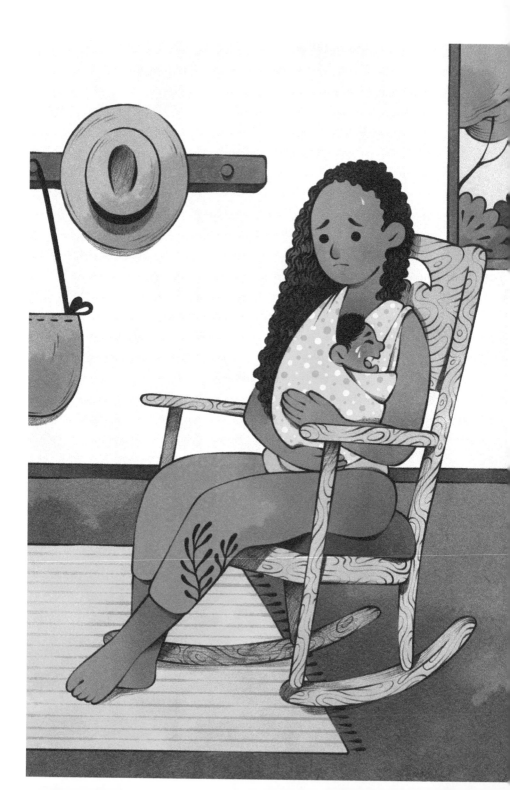

STEP 1:

survive the first three months

YOU READ THE TITLE OF THIS STEP CORRECTLY: Newborns are not actually ready for any sleep training techniques, but that doesn't mean you can't start building healthy sleep habits. Don't panic: There are wonderful things you can do now to move you both in the right direction.

Right now, it's most important to focus on building a bond with your newborn and contributing to his emotional growth. Comfort him, and build trust and security, rather than being firm with any sleep training techniques. At this point, you are following your baby's lead—even though baby's lead might be taking you all over the place!

I know, before you brought your baby home from the hospital, you imagined this cute bundle of joy draped across your chest like in a Pampers Swaddlers commercial. It was the picture of bliss. For some new parents this is reality, but for many parents it's the exact opposite. Let's be real: Newborn sleep is erratic! Completely all over the place, inconsistent, with no pattern whatsoever. One minute your baby looks so peaceful, and the next minute he's bawling. But guess what? That's normal. Let's explore why.

A newborn's stomach is the size of a cherry at birth, a walnut by day three, and an apricot after one week. Although it grows a lot in that first month, it's only the size of an egg by one month of age. This teeny tummy means that a newborn's sleep revolves around the need to eat.

A newborn's sleep patterns are also immature and not yet developed. Newborns aren't equipped with the hormones or sleep cycles necessary for consistent, consolidated, and peaceful sleep. Sure, you may get some longer stretches of sleep at times, but for the most part, you're probably strategizing how to get your newborn to sleep well. You're probably also trying to figure out how to take a shower— or even just a bathroom break—without your baby screaming her head off the moment you lay her down.

I know there's a lot of information out there, but to cut through the myriad of conflicting advice sources on the Internet, I'll try to simplify things by discussing the most important takeaways about newborn sleep. These are the golden rules, and if you do nothing else but follow these guidelines, you should help set your baby on a path to good sleep.

resolve day-night confusion

Newborns are born with an undeveloped circadian rhythm—the 24-hour cycle that dictates sleep and wake patterns. They also don't yet produce much melatonin (the hormone that promotes sleep). And let's not forget that while in the womb, your baby was swayed to sleep during the day—and was often awake at night when you were sleeping (remember those kicks?). For these reasons, babies are often born with their days and nights mixed up. Here are some tips to help reverse your baby's day-night confusion:

LET YOUR BABY KNOW IT'S DAYTIME. Keep the blinds and shades open and allow the light to come in during the day. When nighttime approaches, you'll want to do the exact opposite. Dim the lights, including screens and electronics, during your bedtime routine.

MAKE NOISE DURING THE DAY. Household noise, television, music— this all signals to your baby that it's time to be awake. At night, prior to the bedtime routine, tone down the noise, turn off all distractions, and speak in a quieter, gentler voice. You can even put some relaxing lullabies on low in the background.

LIMIT DAYTIME SLEEP PERIODS. There may be times when your baby does want to sleep a bit longer, as part of that inconsistent and erratic newborn sleep, but it's helpful to intervene a bit. Limit each daytime nap to 2 hours at most; during the evening hours, you may even have to limit it further and only allow catnaps of 30 to 45 minutes. Limiting day sleep also ensures that your baby is getting enough daytime feedings. If he is allowed to nap too long, he may end up with fewer feedings by the end of the day.

RECORD BABY'S SLEEP IN A JOURNAL. Even though sleep at this age is inconsistent, you'll likely find a pattern in the amount of sleep your baby gets in a 24-hour period. This will help you decide how many hours of naptime your baby can get before it starts to interfere with her night sleep. For example, if your baby naps for a total of six hours, and then sleeps a total of eight hours at night, you will likely notice that when she naps for four hours, she sleeps 10 hours at night (with feedings in between, of course). Journaling may help you see this correlation.

calm your baby

Newborns typically cry when they are hungry, wet, or tired. They cycle through these needs and cry periodically throughout the day. Most newborns cry an average of one to two hours per day!

However, there are times when all these needs have been met and baby continues to cry—this is when it starts to get really frustrating for parents. Some babies just have a hard time transitioning to being outside of the womb, because the environment is so different. Here are some ways to help your newborn settle into this big, bright world:

SWADDLE YOUR BABY. I can't stress enough how much difference a swaddle makes for a newborn's sleep. Your baby is used to a very tight, cozy space from when he was in the womb, so suddenly sleeping with his arms and legs free may be a very uneasy feeling for him. A newborn also has a very strong startle reflex; if his uncoordinated arms are left unswaddled, it will be more difficult for your baby to settle to sleep, and this reflex will continue to wake him several times a night. There are hundreds of different swaddles on the market—all with different materials, shapes, and features. These are safer than blankets and very useful for babies' comfort. I recommend conducting your own bit of research to decide which materials, style, and features will work best for your baby.

SAFETY CHECK

✓ Be careful to avoid overheating by making sure your baby is not overbundled in a swaddle. Signs of overbundling include red cheeks, sweating, or skin that is hot to the touch.

✓ For safety reasons, swaddling should be discontinued at the first sign that your baby is ready to roll over. At this point, you can substitute a sleep sack.

✓ Don't force baby's legs down in the swaddle. Allow her hips to spread apart and bend up. According to the International Hip Dysplasia Institute, sudden straightening of the legs can loosen the joints and damage the soft cartilage of the hip socket.

USE WHITE NOISE. This can be extremely helpful. It might be surprising to learn that the womb is a loud environment, so most newborns settle well with a bit of white noise. Some favorite sounds at this age are recordings of womb sounds, a fan, running water, or a vacuum. You may notice that your newborn is immediately interested in these sounds.

ROCK, SWAY, AND BOUNCE YOUR BABY. These all mimic the movements your baby felt in the womb, and often work nicely when combined with the swaddle and white noise.

GO FOR A WALK. There may be times when swaddling, white noise, and other comforting methods do not help. Try taking your baby for a walk in his stroller. The outside air, noise, and even the slightly bumpy ride are often exactly what a newborn needs to settle.

SWITCH OFF WITH A LOVED ONE. A newborn cannot separate your feelings from his, so he may react as if yours are his own feelings—not a good thing when you're feeling stressed. When you are tense, your baby may sense this energy. So if possible, switch off with your partner or get a family member to help—as they say, "it takes a village." What family member or friend wouldn't want to cuddle with a sweet newborn for a little while? You may find that a break from the action is just what you need to feel more calm and relaxed, and as such, have better luck settling your baby.

sleep anywhere?

One of the biggest challenges with newborns is that most of them absolutely hate sleeping flat. This is typically why most babies end up sleeping on Mom or Dad's chest, and then of course will refuse to be put down anywhere else without wailing.

EXTRA HELP: COLIC

Some newborns cry more than average. Colic is defined as crying that persists for more than three hours a day, more than three days a week, for more than three weeks. This crying is typically intense and hard to settle. There are many theories behind this issue, but the true cause of colic is unknown, which can make things even more frustrating when trying to settle a colicky baby. Most colic settles by 3 to 4 months of age. If your baby fits into this category, be sure to talk with your pediatrician. Here are some additional tips:

GET SUPPORT. If your doctor confirms that your baby has colic, ask for and accept the support of your family or friends. Have them stay with your baby while you take a walk, shower, or just leave the house for a little while.

TAKE BREAKS. If you are alone and your baby has been crying and you need a break, lay her down on her back in a safe sleep space, like the crib. Make sure it's bare, free of any suffocation dangers like toys or blankets. Your colicky baby will likely cry whether she is in your arms or in a crib. Laying her down so that you can take a break for a few minutes can help you gather yourself and catch your breath, as holding a crying baby can be extremely hard on your psyche. You should never hold your baby when you feel angry. Instead, put her down in her empty crib and take a break. If the anger persists, call a trusted friend, family member, or doctor for assistance.

TRY SKIN-TO-SKIN CONTACT. There aren't any studies that confirm that this will help with colic, but holding a baby skin to skin has so many other benefits—it helps with bonding, decreases crying, calms baby, and eases the transition out of the womb. You can see why it's definitely worth a try. A baby carrier is another alternative.

CHANGE YOUR ENVIRONMENT. Distractions, such as a change of scenery, can be helpful. Take a walk with your baby in a stroller or baby carrier.

According to the American Academy of Pediatrics and the Safe to Sleep campaign to prevent Sudden Infant Death Syndrome (SIDS), it is dangerous to allow a baby to sleep anywhere other than in a crib. Is it impractical to assume that baby will never nap in your arms? Absolutely! In reality, your baby will likely sleep in a car seat, a swing, a stroller, and yes, in your arms—and undeniably, it feels wonderful. While ideally baby should always sleep in his crib, I will simply emphasize that this is especially true of night sleep, as letting baby sleep in your arms or on your chest can be a very dangerous situation, especially if you are dozing off yourself.

A swing or Rock 'N Play can be a lifesaver, but you should always be cautious with these as well. Most will warn you that they are not intended for unsupervised sleep. During the day, supervising sleep in these devices is easy. But if it is nighttime, and your baby is screaming and absolutely refusing to be laid down in a crib or bassinet, and you cannot hold him because you are falling asleep yourself, then it will be a matter of picking the lesser evil: a screaming baby in a bassinet, or a sleeping baby in a less-than-ideal sleep space like a Rock 'N Play or swing. Deciding which one is a personal choice.

I remember when my first baby was born, she absolutely refused to be laid down flat. She cried so hard that she held her breath and looked like she was turning blue. The only thing she accepted was the Rock 'N Play. Sure, there are definitely safety concerns because of its positioning, but in my opinion, her crying and my sleep deprivation created a much more dangerous situation. I couldn't let her cry like that, and I couldn't hold her because I was afraid I would drop or suffocate her if I fell asleep—and trust me, I was falling asleep! The only viable option was that Rock 'N Play. Neither option was considered safe, but one felt safer than the other. I had to use my mother's intuition and make that call. As days passed, I continued to lay her down in the bassinet at the start of each sleep time, and used the Rock 'N Play as backup. This helped her eventually accept her bassinet.

lay the groundwork

Although newborns are too young for any firm sleep training methods, you can certainly start teaching good sleep habits. A bedtime routine is a great start to forming good habits that can last throughout childhood. A bedtime routine helps cue your baby that it's nearing time to sleep, but it's also a special chance for you and your baby to unwind and connect after a busy day. At this age, the routine should be short and simple; something like feeding, singing a lullaby, and rocking your baby is perfect.

Something else you can get a head start on: practicing laying your baby down awake. Don't assume your baby will only sleep when held. There may be times when you lay your baby down and he'll be content and won't cry—that's good practice! The more practice your baby gets, the more he will accept being laid down in his own cozy sleep space. Once he can do this, sleep typically improves quite a bit. However, at this age, never force this. If your baby is crying, simply comfort him. Remember that this is just practice. Follow your newborn's lead, and he will let you know if he is ready to be laid down awake.

Getting through the newborn stage is often simply a matter of survival—seriously! You are doing what you can as a new parent just to get through this stage, when frequent night wakings, lots of crying (from both you and your baby—it's all okay; we all do it!), and what seem like never-ending feedings are weighing you down. The newborn stage is short and fleeting and so sweet in retrospect, but it can feel like an eternity when you are going through it. I promise it gets better. One day you will look back at this period in your life and laugh at the silly things you did just to get your baby to sleep. I still laugh at all of the times I danced in my kitchen to Alicia Keys with the microwave fan on high, while holding my screaming newborn, who only settled that way. Or how I had to take her on a stroller walk every evening around 5:00 or 6:00 p.m. when the witching hour hit, purposely seeking out and rolling over all of the little bumps in the road because it helped her get calm. In the moment, it was hard to see a light at the end of the newborn tunnel. Looking back, I realize it is a stage we all have to go through. Luckily, it is a very temporary stage.

newborn sleep faq

Q: HOW DO I GET MY NEWBORN TO SLEEP FOR LONGER STRETCHES?

A: Because of her underdeveloped circadian rhythm, your baby's appetite will dictate how long she sleeps. At this stage, you will probably just have to wait it out until her belly grows and matures. In the meantime, speak to your pediatrician about a good feeding schedule. If your baby isn't eating enough during the day, she will likely wake more at night.

Q: MY BABY HATES BEING SWADDLED. WHAT CAN I DO?

A: As a sleep consultant, I hear this often from parents: distraction is key. Once you swaddle your baby, quickly pick him up, rock him, shush in his ear, or put on some white noise in the background. You will see that although your baby initially fusses and squirms, he actually comes to love the swaddle as he sleeps much better in one.

Q: SHOULD I USE A PACIFIER?

A: Pacifiers can be an extremely useful tool for calming a newborn. Studies also show that they reduce the risk of SIDS. But I always tell parents that it is a personal choice since there is some debate on pacifier use. Some pediatricians will recommend holding off giving your baby a pacifier until breastfeeding is well established. Also, some studies show an increased risk of ear infections with pacifier use. So you may want to weigh the pros and cons and make your own educated choice.

Q: WHEN CAN I EXPECT A MORE CONSISTENT SLEEP SCHEDULE?

A: Although some parents will brag that their baby slept through the night at two weeks old, this is not typical, nor is it recommended to let them continue sleeping. Right now, your baby's internal clock is underdeveloped, and her small tummy can only hold so much milk to keep her full during the night. Therefore, it's important that she wakes frequently. You may see a decrease in your baby's erratic sleep around three months of age. Most babies will not settle into a schedule until about four months of age.

Q: HOW MANY NAPS SHOULD MY NEWBORN BE TAKING?

A: Several. There is no guideline for the number of naps in the newborn stage, nor for the length of each nap. Some naps may last 20 minutes, while others last two hours.

STEP 2:

create a sleep-friendly space

ONCE YOU GET PAST THOSE FIRST FEW MONTHS, you can step back a bit and focus on making some simple improvements to your baby's sleep space and routine. A sleep-inducing space can play a big role in improving a baby's sleep. A safe sleep environment is just as crucial. During my consultations, I find that many parents make some common mistakes with their baby's sleep environment. So let's talk about how to set up a safe, sleep-inducing environment.

sleep safely

Never compromise safety just to get your baby to sleep. Teaching a baby good sleep habits will get her sleeping better—not the fancy blanket, sleep positioner, baby lounger, or wedge. Besides, those gadgets are all temporary; teaching good sleep habits lasts a lifetime! Here are my top safe sleep tips:

KEEP THE CRIB TOTALLY BARE EXCEPT FOR A TIGHTLY FITTED SHEET. All toys, bedding, crib bumpers, blankets, or pillows should be removed. Although some bedding sets may come with cute crib bumpers, they pose a suffocation risk and should not be used; in fact, many states have banned the sale of crib bumpers. Crib bumpers were originally created to prevent head entrapment in between slats, but with the new safety regulations, the spaces between slats are so small that this is no longer an issue. Also, parents often think that crib bumpers protect against head bumps or bruises. But these are very minor injuries when compared to the greater risks of suffocation, strangulation, and entrapment.

ALWAYS PLACE BABY ON HER BACK TO SLEEP. Babies are at highest risk when placed on their stomach to sleep.

DON'T USE INFANT SLEEP POSITIONERS AND WEDGES. There isn't any evidence that supports the safety or effectiveness of these products. In fact, there have been reports of injury and death when such products are used, especially in a baby's sleep area.

AVOID PRODUCTS THAT CLAIM THEY REDUCE THE RISK OF SIDS. There is currently no clinical or scientific evidence that shows that any baby products or gadgets prevent or reduce the chance of SIDS. In fact, some even increase the risk.

AVOID OVERHEATING. Don't overdress or overbundle your baby. Check your baby for sweating, red cheeks, or skin that's hot to the touch. These are signs that your baby is too warm.

ROOM SHARE BUT DO NOT BED SHARE. Room sharing reduces the risk of SIDS, but bed sharing can be dangerous. Some risks include suffocation, falls, entrapment, and accidentally rolling over onto your baby. Some parents choose to co-sleep because they enjoy it and some find it convenient, but many do it out of desperation. Although parents can implement methods to decrease the risks associated with co-sleeping, such as laying baby on his back, removing blankets, and avoiding sedatives, there really isn't a way to be fully safe, since we cannot control what our body and brain do while we're asleep. Our consciousness and awareness are decreased, and in certain stages of sleep, muscles are paralyzed, creating a dangerous situation. A great alternative to bed sharing is to keep your baby close by in something like the Arm's Reach Co-Sleeper, which keeps him next to you, but in his own sleep space so he can sleep safely.

set up the bedroom

keep it dark!

» Melatonin is a hormone that helps your baby settle to sleep and stay asleep. Light disrupts melatonin. Making the room pitch black really helps a baby sleep better.

» Ditch that cute night-light and keep the room dark. Trust me on this one. I have even seen babies get disrupted by the small lights on a smoke alarm. You can put a tiny piece of black tape over small lights to avoid this pitfall (don't block the smoke alarm sensors, though!).

» Once your baby's sleep improves, he will be able to fall asleep just about anywhere. Some parents worry, though, that their baby will not be able to fall asleep in daylight when they are out of the house. As your baby's sleep improves, you can allow a little bit of light in if you are worried about this.

keep it quiet!

» It can be hard to avoid daytime noise and outside distractions. White noise, such as that provided by a fan or white noise machine, is a great tool to block out potential disruptions.

» White noise should be a constant sound that doesn't change in pitch or tone. Changes in sound can wake a baby or disrupt her sleep.

» Never put a white noise machine near a baby's ear. White noise acts as a buffer between outside noise and your baby; therefore, it's best to put the white noise machine between your baby and the noise, rather than right next to your baby.

» Use a white noise machine that is safe and approved for babies. Some white noise machines are too loud and can hurt your baby's delicate ears. There isn't enough research to tell us what a safe amount of sound is. We do know that 85 decibels is too much for an adult. We also know that the noise recommendation for a hospital nursery is 50 decibels. Keeping these numbers in mind should help you when shopping for a white noise machine.

» I know they're tempting, but avoid mobiles or anything with lights or music. You want to encourage sleep, not play time. Later we'll talk more about exceptions and when it's appropriate to resort to these devices.

keep it warm, but not hot!

» Keep the room where your baby sleeps at a comfortable temperature for an adult.

» As a rule of thumb, your baby should wear no more than one layer more than an adult would be comfortable in.

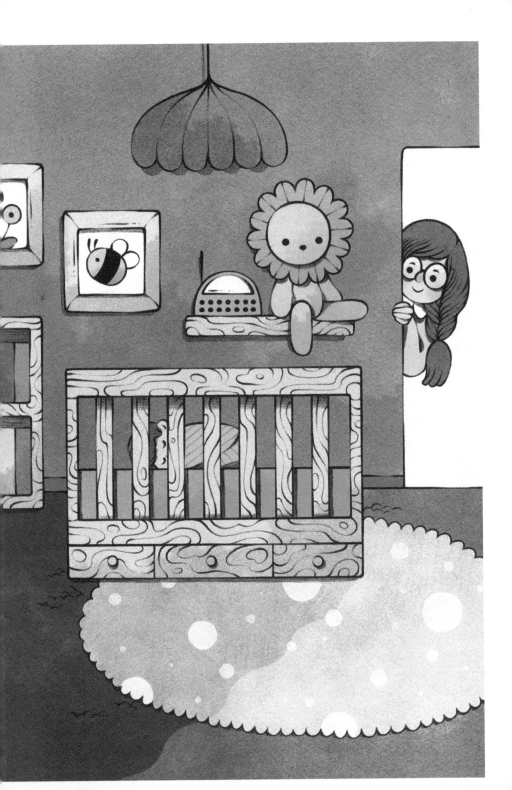

» Ditch the hat! Hospital nurseries put a hat on babies shortly after birth because a newborn baby's head is wet and cold. But this doesn't mean your baby should be sleeping with a hat at home. Hats can cause overheating and can slip off your baby's head onto his face.

» Watch for signs of overheating: red cheeks, a hot chest, and sweating. Overheating increases the risk of SIDS.

get baby used to the crib

During the first couple of months of your baby's life, she has likely spent a lot of time anywhere but the crib. Between the Rock 'N Play naps, swing naps, naps while you are holding her, car seat and stroller naps, getting your baby to actually fall asleep and stay asleep in a crib can be an uphill battle. Here are some suggestions to help ease the transition for a baby who doesn't readily accept the crib:

TAKE BABY STEPS. If your baby is not used to sleeping in a crib, he will likely cry immediately when laid down. So practice laying your baby down a few times a day for a few minutes, or even a few seconds if that is all your baby can handle without crying. Don't give up. The more practice your baby gets, the sooner he will accept the crib.

DISTRACT YOUR BABY. This is a really important tool if your baby's not used to the crib. If you can distract your baby long enough, that's even more practice time in the crib. Now, as I mentioned earlier, I typically don't recommend mobiles with lights or toys, but this is the exception. If you can get your baby to lie down for a few minutes and eventually longer with the use of a mobile, go for it! A mobile can easily be removed once your baby accepts her sleep space.

USE A MIRROR. Babies love staring at their reflection. At a young age they have no idea who they're staring at, but nonetheless, it's very intriguing to them. I have seen many babies doze off while gazing at their reflection, so you may want to try this as another useful distraction tool.

TRY CRIB TIME WHEN YOUR BABY IS MOST CONTENT. It doesn't even have to be naptime, just as long as your baby is content and happy; after a good feeding is a great time. He's more likely to accept the crib when he's not hungry or tired.

PLAY PEEKABOO. This will also distract your baby, as well as help her with object permanence, which develops between four and seven months. If you "disappear" for a few seconds and then reappear, your baby will feel more at ease, knowing you always come back.

QUICK FIX If your baby is having a really hard time falling asleep in the crib, then the goal should not be to sleep in the crib until she is actually willing to *be* in the crib! Instead, try having some fun in there during awake hours. This will help your baby think of the crib as a positive place to be. Lay your baby down as you fold laundry or vacuum, put some music on, and just have fun. Read books, sing some sing-a-long songs, or do anything else that your baby enjoys. Over time, you can reduce the play activities and phase in restful ones, like a sweet bedtime routine.

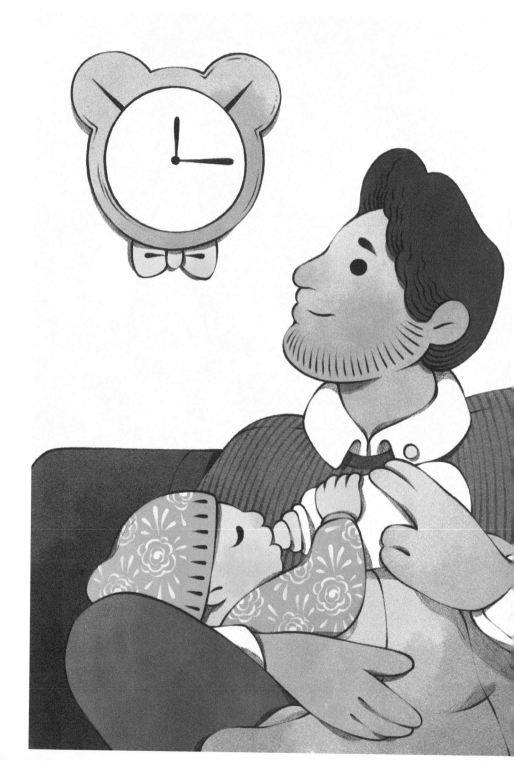

STEP 3:
establish a routine

ESTABLISHING A ROUTINE will help create some predictability in your day. It helps your baby know when certain things are going to happen. A predictable routine decreases anxiety about what's to come, and the end result is a more complaisant baby, especially when it's sleepy time. A typical routine would include feedings in line with your pediatrician's recommended feeding times, some regular fun play or activity time, and then, of course, sleep time, based on your baby's natural rhythm dictating when they need to sleep.

eat, play, sleep

No matter your baby's age, she is in a repetitive cycle of eating, playing, and sleeping throughout the day. Ideally, you want to keep the activities in this order to prevent a feed-to-sleep association, in which a baby expects to be fed right before she goes to sleep. A baby who is fed to sleep typically wakes in between sleep cycles and asks to be fed *back* to sleep. Separating the feeding and sleep with an activity is a smart start to teaching good sleep habits.

Here's a sample of what an eat, play, sleep schedule might look like for a six-month-old:

» 7:00: Awake for the day
» 7:30: Eat
» 8:00–9:00: Play
» 9:30–10:30: Nap 1
» 10:45: Eat
» 11:15 a.m.–12:30 p.m.: Play
» 1:00–2:00: Nap 2
» 2:15: Eat
» 2:45–4:00: Play
» 4:30–5:15: Sleep (catnap)
» 5:30: Eat
» 5:45–6:45: Play
» 7:00: Eat
» 7:15: Bedtime routine
» 7:45: Asleep

Please follow your pediatrician's recommendations for feeding schedules.

QUICK FIX If your baby is waking prematurely from sleep, such as always taking short naps or waking too early in the morning, you may want to add a short activity between waking up and eating: eat, play, sleep, play, then repeat. This will further dissociate feeding from sleep. If baby is waking too early, he may be doing so because he knows that the moment he wakes, he will get his favorite thing in the world: a feeding. But if your baby knows that he will have to do something else first when he wakes, this will encourage him to go back to sleep if he wakes up too early.

recognize drowsy signs

It's important to learn your baby's tiredness signs, so you don't miss her sleepy window: that prime window of opportunity to put your baby down for bed. Putting a baby down to sleep when she's over- or under-tired can result in a teary struggle. The sweet spot for putting your baby down is when she is just starting to get tired, but before she gets overtired. When a baby gets overtired, her body compensates by producing adrenaline. She ends up wired, rather than tired.

Here are some typical sleepy cues:

» Eye rubbing
» Yawning
» Fussiness
» Noises/yelling, or cries that gradually increase in length and frequency
» Decrease in activity
» Loss of interest in playing

set bedtime and wake-up time

Want to set your baby's internal clock? Keep a set bedtime and wake-up time. When a baby goes to sleep and wakes up at about the same times each day, his body starts to produce certain hormones at those times to aid sleep, and wake him up when it's time to get up. This is part of your baby's internal biological clock.

Putting a baby to sleep at 6:30 p.m. one night, and 9:00 p.m. the next night, for example, not only disrupts her internal clock but also makes it very difficult for her to fall asleep and stay asleep. Keeping a consistent bedtime and wake-up time is an important component of improving your baby's sleep.

AGE	NUMBER OF NAPS	NAP SLEEP	NIGHT SLEEP	TOTAL SLEEP
NEWBORN	Several	5–8 hours	Varies	14–17 hours
3 MONTHS	4	2–4 hours	10–12 hours	14–17 hours
6 MONTHS	2–3	2–3.5 hours	10–12 hours	12–15 hours
9 MONTHS	2	2–3 hours	10–12 hours	12–15 hours
12 MONTHS	1–2	2–3 hours	10–12 hours	11–14 hours
18 MONTHS	1	2–3 hours	10–12 hours	11–14 hours
24 MONTHS	0–1	0–2 hours	10–12 hours	11–14 hours

That said, you don't have to obsess over keeping the bedtime exact each night. Up to a 30-minute difference rarely has any impact on sleep. And if your baby occasionally wants to sleep in, like on a cozy Sunday morning, let him! You can adjust by shortening one of his naps.

An ideal bedtime for babies over 3 months old up to toddlerhood is between 7:00 p.m. and 8:30 p.m. An ideal wake-up time is between 6:00 a.m. and 8:30 a.m. Of course, individual variations in schedule may be necessary due to work or other commitments. These are suggested bedtimes and wake-up times in an ideal world. We all know that ideal is not always possible, and that's fine. Follow these times if they work for you, and if you can't, just adjust to your family's schedule.

Newborns don't really follow set bedtimes and wake-up times, since they have immature and underdeveloped internal clocks. Their bedtime tends to be late, since they have a hard time settling for bed in the early evening. This is a phenomenon known as the "witching hour." It is not unusual for newborns to settle after 9:00 or 10:00 p.m., and sometimes even later. Don't stress, and don't try to force your newborn to fall asleep early; just follow her lead. Over time, you'll notice that your baby will start to accept an earlier bedtime. Somewhere between three and four months of age, your baby should settle into a bedtime of around 8:00 or 8:30 p.m.

create a bedtime routine

Bedtime routines are a wonderful opportunity for both you and your baby to relax, unwind, and bond. They are also important signals to your baby that bedtime is coming. When your baby knows what's coming, she will be much less apprehensive. Some babies even look forward to the bedtime routine. Here are some things to keep in mind when creating a bedtime routine:

HAVE FUN! Your routine should be enjoyable for both you and your baby. Include things like lullabies, bedtime books, cuddling, or anything else both you and your baby enjoy.

NOT TOO SHORT, NOT TOO LONG. With a short routine, your baby won't have enough time to unwind. A routine that is too long may disinterest your baby. An ideal routine is 20 to 25 minutes long, or 10 to 15 minutes for a newborn up to three months old.

KEEP IT SIMPLE. I always tell parents that the routine should be simple enough that when you are not home for bedtime, you can still implement some of the activities to help cue your baby to sleep. If your bedtime routine is very elaborate, it may be hard to replicate it on the go. This may discourage you from going out, and you deserve an occasional night out past bedtime!

KEEP BATH TIME SEPARATE FROM THE BEDTIME ROUTINE. I typically don't consider bath time a part of the bedtime routine. For one, most babies don't need a bath every single night. Bathing your baby every night just for the sake of routine is not very practical, and you will drive yourself nuts trying to implement this every night! You should have a sufficient routine (20 to 25 minutes) that does not include bathing. Second, consider the times when you are out at dinner or a friend's house, and can't give your baby a bath. As above, keep it simple for success!

EXTRA HELP: GOING OUT

You *can* go out and stay out past bedtime. Making sure you are home at 7:00 p.m. every night will put a huge strain on your social life, and you just don't need to be that firm. Your baby will be fine if she stays up past her bedtime occasionally, or falls asleep in the car on the way home. If you know that you'll be out late, bring your baby's pjs, make sure she has her last feeding, use a key phrase to cue sleep, such as "it's sleepy time," and lay her down anywhere you are. When you get home, just transfer your baby to the crib; no need to go through the bedtime routine again.

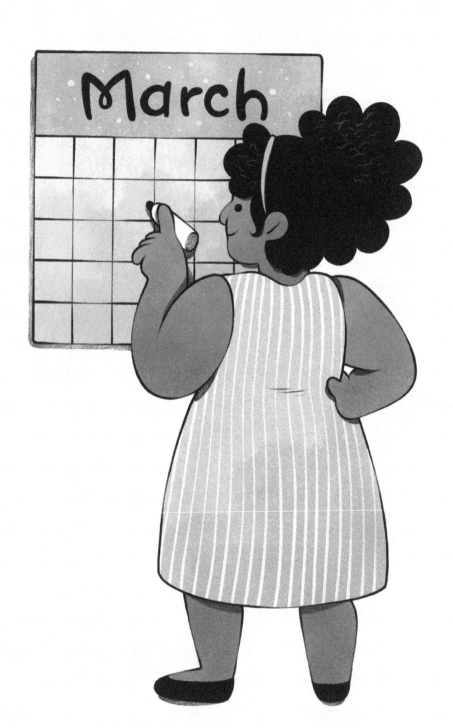

STEP 4:
choose your moment

CHOOSING THE RIGHT TIME to sleep train can be as difficult as deciding on the best time to go on vacation with a baby. As much as you think you have it figured out, there will never be a 100 percent perfect time. And inevitably something always comes up, but you don't necessarily cancel your vacation plans! The same goes with sleep training—there will never be a perfect time, but there may be a time that is better.

Once you decide on a time, clear your calendar and prepare yourself with all the information I'm about to give you. It will help you know what to do, when to do it, and how to stay positive even if you experience challenges.

decide when you're ready

Not every baby needs sleep training. Some babies are just born good sleepers. Yes, this may be hard to believe, but a small percentage of babies learn to sleep well all by themselves. Some babies can be rocked, fed, or held to sleep, and then sleep fine the rest of the night. If your baby sleeps well, and you don't see a problem with your baby's sleep, then you may not have to sleep train at all. Don't feel like you have to sleep train just because others are—you may just have a very good sleeper on your hands, and that's enviable!

Most babies who do need sleep training have become reliant on sleep props like rocking, swinging, car rides, mobiles, bouncing, or feeding to sleep. Whether or not a baby needs to be sleep trained often depends on his sensitivity to these sleep props. A baby who is sensitive to sleep props (true of most babies) will rely on that prop to fall asleep, and will then wake several times a night wanting the prop because he doesn't know any other way to get back to sleep. If this describes your baby, he will most likely need some sleep training to help resolve these sleep troubles.

Here are some signs that your baby is ready for sleep training:

» Your baby is at least five months old.

» Your baby is waking several times a night and needs assistance getting back to sleep.

» Your baby is waking frequently and not getting enough sleep.

» Your baby is constantly tired and cranky and looks like she needs more sleep.

» Her naps are poor, short, and often a struggle.

» You find yourself rocking, holding, or feeding for extended periods at sleep times, and have to do it all over again after your baby wakes when laid down.

EXTRA HELP: PARENT SLEEP

Naturally, when your baby isn't sleeping, neither are you. You're tired, irritable, and at your wit's end. The smallest of tasks seems daunting. And instead of having fun with your baby, you feel like he's torturing you. In other words, you're not feeling at your parenting best.

A recent study showed that when you aren't getting enough sleep or have been awake for too many hours, your cognitive and motor performance is equivalent to that of a drunk person! Getting some decent zzz's is important for both your physical and emotional well-being. The best thing you can do right now for you and your baby is encourage good sleep habits by sleep training. You may want to get your partner to help out while you catch up on some sleep first, or alternate nights during the sleep-training process. You can also enlist your village—call on family and friends to help so you can get a nap during the day. Lastly, try to get to bed as soon as your baby does. Often the first stretch of baby's night sleep is the longest, so take advantage!

» Your baby continues to struggle with sleep.

» Your pediatrician or health advisor believes your baby no longer needs night feedings, but your baby is still waking.

avoid troubled times

There's never really a "perfect" age to sleep train. There will always be bumps in the road and new developments that can make sleep training challenging—growth spurts, baby's urge to practice new skills, and separation anxiety are just a few. Just because these developments exist, though, does not mean you should have to postpone sleep training. If you wait until nothing is going on, you may *never* get a chance to sleep train! With all of the changing, growing, and developing your baby goes through, there will ALWAYS be something going on. But by equipping him with good sleep habits, you will help him breeze through these bumps without a hitch.

In my work as a sleep consultant, parents often report that once they've implemented my sleep training program, they no longer notice their baby going through any major bumps or regressions. Once babies learn to sleep well, they have those skills in place to help them be better sleepers through challenging times. This is another excellent reason to sleep train.

Of course, you'll want to be mindful of certain milestones and stages in your baby's development, so that you can offer extra comfort, love, and attention during these times. But don't avoid sleep training completely, because in my experience, sleep troubles escalate over time. The only time I really don't recommend sleep training is when your baby is sick or uncomfortable, simply because it wouldn't be fair to expect your baby to sleep well if she isn't feeling well.

WHEN SHOULD I SLEEP TRAIN?	NO SLEEP TRAINING	MAYBE	GREAT AGE	TRICKY AGE
0 TO 2 MONTHS	X			
3 TO 4 MONTHS		X		
5 TO 7 MONTHS			X	
8 TO 10 MONTHS				X
11 TO 12 MONTHS				X
18 TO 24 MONTHS				X

The chart on the previous page shows the best and trickiest times to sleep train, and the subsequent list describes some of the pros and cons of sleep training at each age. Please note that just because your baby is at a tricky age to sleep train (such as eight months and older) does not mean you should avoid it. Go ahead and start, so you can prevent those bad sleep habits from becoming more embedded and increasingly difficult to conquer.

0 to 2 months

» Baby is too young for any formal sleep training. Instead, focus on the tips in the "Survive the First Three Months" section.

» It can take a baby six to eight weeks for day-night confusion to resolve.

» A baby's sleep-wake cycle doesn't start to develop until six weeks of age. By three to six months, most infants have a regular sleep-wake cycle.

» Your baby won't start producing enough melatonin to sleep well until about two to three months. Before this age, getting to sleep and staying asleep might take some effort.

» Your baby will also hit the first three growth spurts during this time (one week, three weeks, and six weeks). This may mean more feedings and more wakings.

3 to 4 months

» Baby may be ready for some gentle sleep training as long as it doesn't result in crying. Focus on comfort rather than letting him cry. If your baby accepts the techniques without crying, great! If he doesn't, try again in a few weeks.

» The first sleep regression happens during this period. When a baby is learning a new skill (like rolling over), he's going to want to practice even at night, which may keep him up. Lots of practice time during the day helps.

» Baby will also hit the three-month growth spurt during this stage.

5 to 7 months

» This is a great age for sleep training. Your baby is far past the newborn stage, he is more mobile so he can get into a comfy sleep position, and many experts agree that most babies don't need nighttime feedings by six months of age. (Please check with your pediatrician.)

» Babies love to practice sitting and other skills, especially when you lay them down to sleep. This will pass once your baby has mastered the skill.

» Be aware of the six-month growth spurt, which can disrupt sleep.

8 to 10 months

» This is a tricky age for sleep training, but don't postpone it. Instead, offer extra comfort if necessary.

» Crawling often causes a second sleep regression. Babies love practicing their emerging skills, such as crawling, at bedtime and even in their sleep.

» Object permanence is developed, which means your baby knows something exists even when it's not in sight. So when she wakes up at night, she may miss you and start looking for you.

» Separation anxiety starts to peak. Some nights, it may be hard for your baby to fall asleep and stay asleep, especially when you come back from a party or event where your baby was around many unfamiliar faces.

» There will be times when you go to lay your baby down, and up he stands! No guilt necessary, Moms and Dads; this is just practice, not desperation! Your baby may practice this skill over and over until he masters it.

11 to 12 months

» Babies can be distracted by language development. They may be thinking of words they have learned and practicing them in their little heads when they should be sleeping. (Kind of like us, right?)

» Another common sleep regression happens at 12 months. Babies are going through tremendous physical development as they learn to walk and even climb. This can definitely carry over into sleep time.

18 to 24 months

» At this age, your baby enjoys testing you. Now that she is discovering that what she does has a direct effect on your reaction, she may start to refuse naps and bedtime, just to see what you'll do.

» Due to this testing behavior, it can be a struggle to sleep train, but I definitely still recommend it, as long-term sleep issues can linger if not addressed.

clear your calendar

Like with anything, sleep training is most successful when you have time to dedicate to it. Here are some factors to consider:

START ON A WEEKEND. Often the first few nights are the hardest, so I recommend sleep training over a weekend if you have work or other commitments during the week. It will make the process less stressful if you know that you don't have to wake up early or be somewhere by a certain time.

POSTPONE SLEEP TRAINING IF YOU HAVE IMMEDIATE TRAVEL PLANS. The last thing you want to do is put in all of this hard work sleep training and then regress when inevitably, your baby sleeps worse during travel. Once your baby is sleep trained, traveling will be a breeze. But for now, while you are laying the foundation of good sleep habits, it is best to avoid travel.

DON'T PLAN ANY PLAY DATES. Baby classes, play dates, and other fun activities that run into sleep time should be avoided during the first week of sleep training to keep the schedule consistent. These activities can also overstimulate your baby and make it more difficult for her to fall asleep. The first week is often the most crucial, when you are building a foundation of good sleep habits. If you have a choice, it's even better to further solidify this by taking a second week off from activities.

prepare for the seven days

WE'RE CLOSING IN ON THE BIG WEEK! You can set yourself up for success by preparing a few last things ahead of time. Set up the nursery to promote a sleep-friendly environment. Get everyone on board (partner, grandma, nanny, etc.) to make sure your team is consistent in its efforts. Chat with your pediatrician about sleep training. You may even want to talk to your baby's daycare folks and see how open they are to implementing some of the same sleep-time regimens you're planning at home.

Next, we'll talk about setting a goal for this sleep training, having a plan in mind, and always remembering why you are doing this in the first place: so you can have a happy and well-rested baby and be a happy and well-rested parent.

set a goal

Think about what you want your sleep goal to be, and ask yourself if the goal is realistic. Are you okay with one to two feedings a night? Is your goal to decrease wakings? Do you want to stop rocking for over an hour every night? Keeping your goal in mind will help set clear expectations and make your goal more attainable. It's important to pick a measurable goal, so it's easier to see if you're making progress.

Here are some examples of realistic and measurable sleep training goals:

FEWER WAKINGS. Any decrease in wakings is progress, right? If you can get a baby who was waking four times a night to wake only two times a night, for example, that's a great change, and it's very attainable. Realistic goals put less pressure on both you and your baby, and give you hope that you can make additional progress in the future using the same plan.

LESS PROTESTING AT SLEEP TIMES. As your baby gets used to her routine, she will start to accept it. When she starts to accept it, she won't cry or protest as much, and eventually she will not fuss at all. A goal to decrease opposition to sleep time is very realistic.

SHORTENED TRANSITION TO SLEEP. When a baby isn't sleeping well, has bad sleep habits, or has a sleep schedule that's all over the place, he typically takes quite a while to fall asleep at bedtime. As you work to change your baby's sleep habits, you should notice that your baby falls asleep faster and more easily. This is a great goal to aim for!

LESS ASSISTANCE TO SLEEP. If you are working on helping your baby fall asleep on her own, decreasing the amount of help you give her is a great goal. If you had been rocking her for over 45 minutes, but now she's falling asleep in only 15 minutes, that's a huge accomplishment and was a very attainable goal.

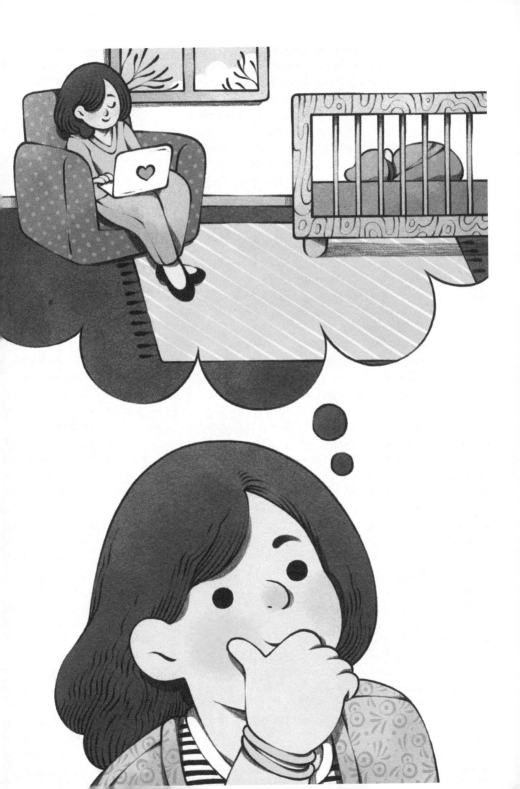

QUICK FIX Of all the sleep training goals, I find that parents get the most frustrated with the task of decreasing the amount of assistance they give their baby at sleep time. There's a misconception that parents have to lay their baby down awake on the first night, and baby has to fall asleep on his own. However, independent sleep is a process, and it may take a few nights before you can even lay your baby down without major hysterics. Try to keep it real, even if you are exhausted and desperate for change. Setting a goal that is too difficult will leave you throwing in the towel before you even have a chance to see that it does get better. As you begin the process, try to remember that a realistic goal, like decreasing the amount of assistance you are giving your baby to sleep, is much more attainable than aiming for your baby to fall asleep on his own right away.

make a plan

A consistent plan is often the key to sleep training success. In the next section, "During the Seven Days," I will provide you with just that: a consistent plan to follow. This plan is a guide; by all means, make alterations to fit your family's goals. However, be sure to plan out those alterations ahead of time so you can remain as consistent as possible. Consistency will ensure that baby knows what to expect, and will decrease the tears. It will also speed progress.

get on the same page

If you are working on the plan with a partner, it is important that you are both on the same page and being consistent. Inconsistencies can make the process very frustrating. For example, if Dad is working really hard at not feeding the baby to sleep, then Mom goes in

EXTRA HELP: SIBLINGS

Parents often worry about waking up a sibling during sleep training, especially if the two children share a room. In my experience, most siblings aren't as bothered by this as parents might anticipate. Also, this sort of disruption is very short-lived. In a few nights, everyone should be sleeping much better. A fear of waking the family often prolongs the sleep training, and sometimes even deters it altogether. The problem with putting things off is that the wakings typically don't stop, so the family is getting even more disruption in the long run than they would have with a few nights of sleep training—just think five-year-old insisting on sleeping in your bed ev-er-y night! Don't let the fear of waking others stop you from teaching your little one good sleep habits. Of course, if you have an option of sleep training in a different bedroom, you can certainly do that. If you don't, don't worry, everyone will survive, and ultimately thrive!

and feeds her to sleep, that just erased all of Dad's hard work. Talk in advance about how to handle situations like this, so you're able to stay consistent and make the process go more smoothly.

Here are some things to discuss:

» Who will handle bedtime?

» Who will handle the night wakings? Should we alternate?

» Exactly how are we handling the night wakings?

» What's our Plan B if a night waking is taking a really long time?

» When do we take a break?

» When do we call it quits for the night?

✓ Now is a good time to speak to your pediatrician about sleep training. Give her an outline of what you intend to do, to be sure she's okay with it. It is also very important to discuss night feedings with your pediatrician or health advisor before attempting to night-wean. They know how your baby is growing and gaining, and if he still needs to eat at night. However, just because your baby still needs a night feeding or two does not mean that you cannot teach healthy sleep habits. We'll explore how to do this once we dive into the seven-day plan. In the meantime, knowing what to do about night feedings is important so you'll know exactly how to handle a night waking and avoid unnecessary crying when your baby is hungry. If you feel your baby is hungry at any point during the sleep training, you should go ahead and feed.

know what you're capable of

It can be challenging as a new parent to teach a baby to sleep well. You're basically changing your baby's routine and replacing it with a new one. Think of it as one of your first opportunities to take the lead—you're the parent now. Oh yes, your baby will likely be upset about these new changes. And since a baby's only way of communicating is crying, she will likely cry to let you know how unhappy she is about this. Crying is what parents struggle with the most when it comes to sleep training. Understandably so—no one wants to hear their baby cry! But when you understand *why* your baby is crying, it can make the process much easier. Crying is not always a sign of distress. Babies cry to convey a wide range of emotions during sleep training, including frustration, overstimulation, anger, overtiredness, or just plain dissatisfaction. Our job as parents is not always to stop the crying at any cost. Sometimes our job is to just listen and wholeheartedly provide love and support, even if there's a bit of crying.

I like to use the following example: If your baby or toddler wants to eat chocolate cake for breakfast, lunch, and dinner, would you let him just to avoid his heartbreaking cries? Or would you say "no," because it's not healthy, and deal with the waterworks? Sleep training should be looked at the same way. Frequent night wakings and inadequate sleep are no healthier than eating chocolate cake all day. So saying "no" to the bad sleep habits is necessary, even if your baby is upset about it. It will be the first of many times that you as a parent will make the unpopular decision, and it's okay!

There may be times when you think that there is *no way* that this is going to work. There will likely be nights when you want to give up. One of the most common mistakes I see parents make is deciding way too early that the sleep training is not working. They don't get to see the shift; that it *does* get better. Your baby needs time to get used to the new routine. Give your little one a fair chance—for you and for her. You will be amazed at how quickly she can learn. When she does, you'll see an improvement in sleep and you'll catch that first glimpse of hope. Don't mistake that for luck; it's your hard work. Stay strong and don't let one bad night get you down, because healthy, peaceful, and restful sleep for the entire family is so worth the journey getting there.

during the seven days

Get your parenting pants on, your positive spirit at the ready, and your goals in hand, and prepare to take the first steps toward healthy sleep habits for everyone. It's time to sleep train, and we'll walk through each step of the process so you can handle this without breaking a sweat.

1 **put baby to bed**

2 **check in**

3 **stay strong**

4 **handle night wakings**

5 **repeat**

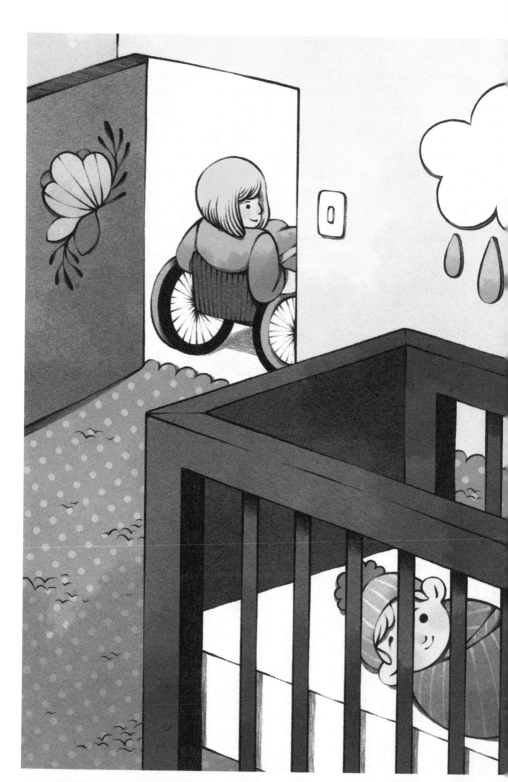

STEP 1:

put baby
to bed

IT'S DAY ONE OF SLEEP TRAINING, and you're ready to get started. The first step is just putting your baby to bed, but it's a more important step than you might think. How you put your baby to sleep is one of the most vital aspects of teaching her to sleep well. This often sets the tone for how the rest of the night will go. If your baby is fed, rocked, held, or swayed all the way to sleep, you can expect that she will wake in between sleep cycles asking for the same environment in which she fell asleep. After all, that's how she was taught!

Since babies have many short sleep cycles, this results in frequent night wakings. You'll want to make sure your baby goes down awake so she can fall asleep on her own—this will encourage her to do the same during the night. Keep in mind, independent sleep is an evolution, so don't get discouraged if this doesn't happen right away.

follow your bedtime routine

Now that you've learned how to create a proper bedtime routine (page 26), you can put that routine into action. Remember, the routine should be simple, an appropriate length, and fun!

Since we will be working on independent sleep, your routine should not involve anything that is going to help your baby to sleep. The purpose of sleep training is to teach your baby to fall asleep on her own, but the routine helps keep the message clear that bedtime is coming. If you are rocking or swaying your baby, she's likely to get sleepy, but when you try to lay her down awake, chances are she's going to get quite upset, as she had hopes of you rocking her all the way to sleep. Keeping the message clear by putting her down awake usually results in a much better outcome and fewer tears.

If your baby falls asleep while feeding, move the feeding to the beginning of the bedtime routine. I find that when babies aren't getting a clear message, that's what really ramps up the crying.

put baby down awake

After the last step of your bedtime routine, you are going to lay your baby down awake. Yes, awake! We now know that assisting a baby to sleep typically leads to frequent night wakings. Also, if your baby falls asleep in your arms, then wakes in between sleep cycles in his crib, this can be quite alarming for him. Just imagine if you fell asleep in your bed, but woke up in your backyard. Quite frightening! Such a scare can even make it difficult to calm your baby. Laying your baby down awake so he is aware of his surroundings, even if he is initially upset about it, sets him up for success.

Once you lay your baby down awake, say a consistent key phrase like "it's sleepy time, good night." This phrase will help cue your baby that it's time to sleep. It's also a good verbal reminder that you can use during middle-of-the-night wakings.

leave the room

After you say your key phrase, leave the room. You're not abandoning your baby—you can go back in at any time. It's important to give your baby a fair chance to figure out how to fall asleep without your help. You may be surprised at how fast your baby falls asleep on her own, if just given the opportunity to do so.

EXTRA HELP: A GRADUAL APPROACH

You may be reluctant to leave your baby after the bedtime routine, especially if he has never slept alone or is used to sleeping with you. An alternative to this step is to park a chair beside your baby's crib, but still allow your baby to self-settle. On the first night, you can stay until your baby is fully asleep. On night two or three, you can leave when your baby is very sleepy. Over the next few nights, you are going to want to leave the room as your baby is more and more awake, since you are working toward independent sleep. Within a week—longer if you feel necessary—you should leave after you complete your bedtime routine and lay your baby down so he can fall asleep on his own, without needing your presence.

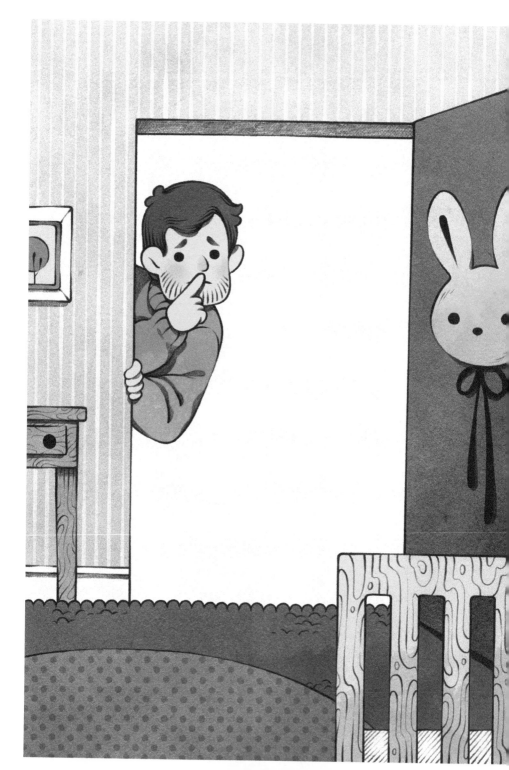

STEP 2:
check in

AFTER YOU'VE LEFT THE ROOM, you'll be giving your baby the time she needs to fall asleep on her own. However, it's important to plan out how often you'll go back in to check on her and what you'll do during these checks. There are two ways to handle check-ins: You can either comfort your baby or just go in for verbal reassurance. Both options let your baby know that you're always nearby, but that she is expected to fall asleep on her own. You will know which works best for your baby based on her response to you. If your baby enjoys the comforting and is still able to settle to sleep on her own, then great; comforting will work well. If your baby's cries intensify, or your comforting makes things worse, then verbal reassurance like shushing and using your key phrase may work best.

decide on an interval

Choosing how long to wait in between checks is dependent on a few different factors. The first you can judge by listening carefully to your baby's cry. If your baby is just fussy or whiny, and you can see that he is safe on a monitor, there's no need to intervene. Your baby is figuring out how to fall asleep unassisted. Think of this as your baby learning a new skill; he's going to get frustrated until he figures it out—just like when he's learning to roll over, crawl, or stack blocks. Fussing, whining, and even some tantrums are part of the learning process. Allow him to do this and resist the urge to go in.

If he really starts crying, start a waiting interval. When deciding how long this interval should be, consider what you are comfortable with. Every family is different, so this factor will vary. For some, two minutes is agony, but for others 10 minutes is no big deal. As a sleep consultant working with so many different families, I understand how individual this part can be. You know your baby best. In my experience, it isn't necessary to commit to a set interval—the important thing is just to commit to *something* so you are giving your baby a fixed opportunity to learn to self-settle. The more consistent practice you can deposit into the independent sleep piggy bank, the quicker your baby will learn to fall asleep on her own.

Finally, your interval may differ from night to night. At times your baby may be completely content, only fussing every so often for 15 to 20 minutes, allowing you to comfortably refrain from going in. Other times you may have to go in after only two minutes because your baby is crying hysterically. As long as you make sure your baby falls asleep on his own, you can go in for a check at any interval that you feel is best.

check in for comfort

If you decide that your baby enjoys comforting and is settled by your touch, then the best strategy is to comfort your baby during check-ins but step out of the room before he's asleep, so your baby can still practice falling asleep on his own.

Comforting includes anything that helps settle your baby. Ideally, you want to start with things that involve the least assistance, then pick her up as a last resort. For example, perhaps first walk in and offer verbal reassurance; if that doesn't work, try some back or belly rubs. If touch in the crib is not helping, then pick her up and rock her. Here's an example of how this might work:

I lay baby down awake.

I say key goodnight phrase and leave the room.

Baby is only fussing. I'm staying away.

Baby is starting to cry. I wait 5 minutes.

I go in and provide comfort until my baby calms down:
Key goodnight phrase » Shushing » Back rubs »
Baby calmed (but still awake)

I leave baby in crib awake, saying key goodnight phrase,
and leave the room.

I repeat these steps until baby falls asleep.

The purpose of the comforting is to help calm your baby enough so she can practice falling asleep on her own. Resist the temptation to comfort your baby all the way to sleep. Otherwise, you'll have just replaced one prop with another.

check in verbally

Some babies will not accept comforting—it's like they're saying, "If you are not going to give me what I want, don't bother with anything else." In this case, going in at intervals just to check on your baby and offer verbal reassurance may work best. If you are opting for this method, it is likely because comforting and touch made your baby more upset, or he expected that you would comfort him all the way to sleep. You can see if a hand on his back or belly will help calm him, but it may be best to simply use your voice in these check-ins.

When you check in verbally, you can offer a key phrase or some shushing as reassurance for your baby that you have not left him, but he still has to fall asleep on his own. The check-ins will also give you peace of mind, since you can see that nothing is wrong, and your baby is just protesting.

A baby camera can provide additional reassurance and allow you to monitor your baby. This tool can help parents remain confident in refraining from entering the room prematurely or when it's not necessary to do so. If your baby is only fussing, and you can visualize that he is safe, you'll be more likely to stay away and allow him to self-settle. Without a camera, you may be inclined to go in more frequently to keep checking on him, but this disturbs the self-settling process.

If you choose verbal checks after comforting checks don't work, you should notice that there is less overall crying than when you tried comforting. The crying may be more intense initially, but will usually subside in half the time.

EXTRA HELP: PERSISTENT CRYING

Some strong-willed babies or babies who are very dependent on help to get to sleep will cry intensely when laid down awake, and no amount of soothing helps. This can be so hard for parents to handle that they have a hard time continuing the sleep training. An alternative to this is to continue using baby's favorite sleep prop, whether that's rocking or even feeding to sleep as a last resort, and phase it out gradually over several nights, making sure baby is more and more awake each night when laid down.

If at any point the crying is too much for your comfort, you can stop and try again at the next waking, or even the next night. You know your baby best. So if you have given the check-ins good effort, but need to stop because the crying is more than what you are comfortable with, please don't feel like you have failed. Often, delaying gratification alone is enough to stop the wakings. In other words, your baby will not want to work that hard for a sleep prop each night, and will eventually accept going to sleep without it. It will likely take longer to see progress than if you just withheld the prop altogether, but of course this is always an option if you are not comfortable with the amount of crying.

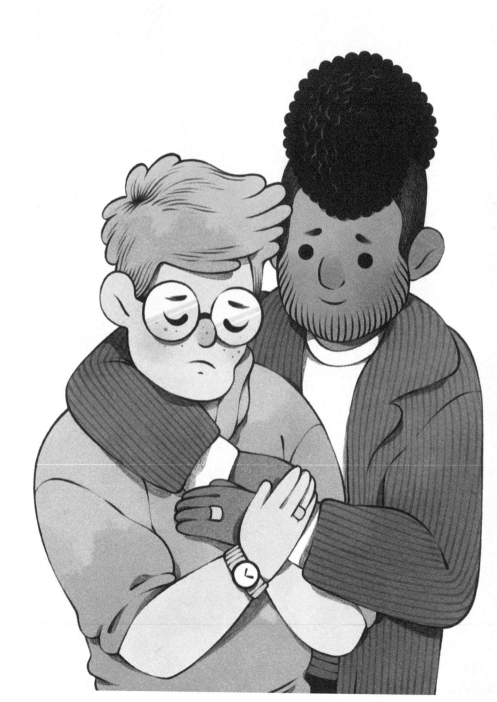

STEP 3:
stay strong

AS YOU START this seven-day sleep training plan, always keep in mind your ultimate goal: to have a happy and well-rested baby, and for you to finally get some zzz's too! Sleep is important for the physical, emotional, and mental health of both you and your baby. Let's explore this a bit—perhaps it'll provide some good motivation if you're feeling challenged.

Sleep is essential for proper growth and development. During the deep stages of sleep, our bodies are busy releasing growth hormones, increasing blood supply to muscles, growing and repairing tissues, and restoring energy to the brain and body. When sleep is disturbed or fragmented, the body doesn't reach enough of these deep stages to complete this process. What does this translate to? A tired, cranky baby, and parents who lack the energy to take care of that baby! Lack of sleep can also impair judgment and decrease awareness. So not only does disturbed sleep feel crummy, but it's also a dangerous situation.

When sleep training gets tough, think about why you are doing it in the first place. When you remind yourself that you are doing this with your baby's best interests at heart, you can never go wrong.

stick to the plan

As we've discussed, don't back down. It's important to stick to the plan so you have a chance to see that it does get better. Immediate improvement is rare; that would be too easy! And sometimes things get worse before they get better. But here are some tips to help you stay the course when things get challenging:

IF YOUR BABY CRIES TOO MUCH FOR YOUR LIKING, TAKE A QUICK BREAK. Take your baby out of the room and restart. Sometimes that little distraction is all you both need. You don't need to start the bedtime routine all over again, just calm down and then get back to laying your baby down awake.

STAY REALISTIC: SLEEP TRAINING TAKES TIME. As a matter of fact, expect the first few nights to be a mess! Sleep always gets worse before it gets better, in part because for the last several weeks or months you may have been exhausting your energy on just maintaining the status quo. Now you are changing your baby's routine, starting a new one, and sticking to it even if it gets tough. Good for you!

WATCH FOR SIGNS OF IMPROVEMENT. Most babies fall asleep on their own within 60 to 90 minutes on the first night, and in about 45 minutes the next. From there, you should see significant improvement between nights three and five. Note that these estimates aren't crying time—I don't recommend that a baby cry for 90 minutes straight! This is just referring to the amount of time it should take your baby to fall asleep on her own. Yes, there may be some crying during this time, but there should also be some quiet periods, comforting, or even taking a break as mentioned.

TRY AGAIN AT THE NEXT WAKING. If at any point your baby is crying more than you are comfortable with, stop and try again at the next waking or the next night. It's worth repeating that you know your baby best.

take care of yourself

SWITCH OFF WITH YOUR PARTNER. When the crying gets tough, switch with your partner or a trusted family member. Your baby may even settle much more easily with them.

KEEP YOUR GOAL IN MIND. Think about why you are doing this in the first place and the goal you set with this sleep training. There's a reason you wanted to do this. Refer back to my chocolate cake example (page 43)!

TAKE NAPS WHEN YOUR BABY NAPS. I know, there's so much laundry to do, but it will be there waiting for you when you wake up feeling better. And since the first few nights will likely be messy with lots of wakings, you will lose some sleep. If you can grab a nap during the day, this will help replenish your energy (another reason to start this plan on a weekend!).

GET HELP FROM FAMILY AND FRIENDS. It's a priceless gift if someone can come over for an hour or two for a few days to help with the baby while you nap. If you're more rested, you'll feel better able to handle the tough first few nights.

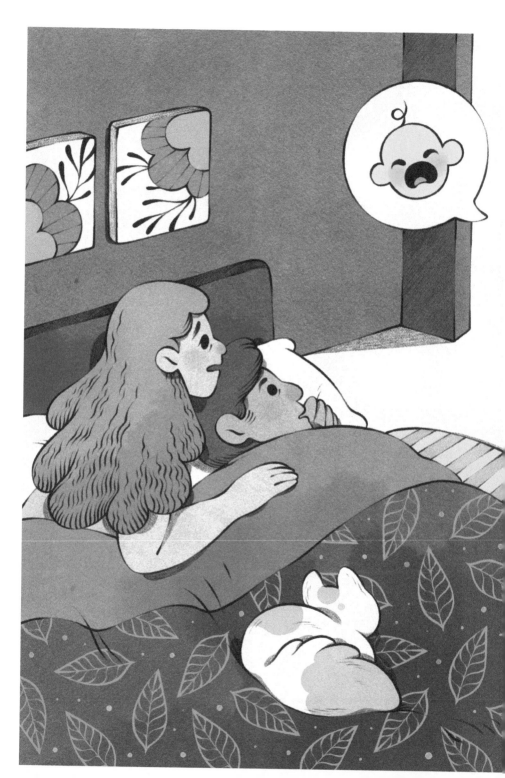

STEP 4:
handle night wakings

YAY, YOU DID IT! Your baby is asleep! But now what? Perhaps you are anxiously waiting for her to wake up screaming. The first few nights she may just do this to see if you're really serious about this whole independent sleep thing. To keep things consistent, you will want to handle the night wakings in a very similar way to bedtime. Here's what you need to know.

when to stay away

When your baby wakes, it is very important to give her enough time to figure out how to fall asleep without your help. Delaying your intervention is the single most important part of nipping night wakings in the bud. Often, if given enough time, a baby will fall back asleep on her own. Once she does that, her sleep will typically improve dramatically, even to the point of sleeping through the night shortly thereafter.

How long you wait before you intervene depends on the same factors we discussed earlier (see page 51), but it should be at least three to five minutes. This is how long it takes a baby to fully awaken and even realize she's awake. Intervening before this time may actually fully awaken your baby, and at that point it will be difficult for her to go back to sleep. Giving your baby enough time will help you confirm she is fully awake, and not just transitioning in between sleep cycles.

It's not unusual for a baby who is first learning to sleep independently to cry out in his sleep, and then drift back to sleep. Waiting to intervene also gives your baby a fair chance to practice going back to sleep on his own. Now, you are probably thinking: "You want me to wait until my baby completely wakes up before going to him?" Yes, absolutely! Remember we are working on independent sleep, meaning we want your baby to fall asleep on his own at bedtime and subsequently during the night. We are no longer "maintaining"; we are full-on working to teach your baby to sleep on his own. This means if he wakes, we want him to go back to sleep unassisted.

Going in too early is the number-one mistake parents make during night wakings. I totally understand this—I've done it myself! You want to quickly run in there before your baby fully wakes so everyone can just drift back to sleep. But this is often what starts the sleep troubles in the first place. Your baby has not learned how to transition in between sleep cycles on her own and keeps waking and expecting you to do it for her. If you keep fearing that your baby will wake, scream, and not go back to sleep, these wakings will just continue. Now is the time to work on this. Be strong—you've got this!

when to intervene

There may be times when you will want to intervene, like when your baby is crying too hard or too much for your liking, and that is perfectly fine. You can go in and check on your baby using the same approach as you did at bedtime. As long as your baby goes back to sleep on his own, you can check on him as you see fit, keeping in mind the principle of giving your baby enough time to practice independent sleep.

Depending on your baby's age, growth, or stage of development, you may need to feed your baby at night. Please check with your pediatrician on how many feedings your baby should get, if any, and how often you should feed. Knowing this information ahead of time is helpful so you'll know exactly how to handle a waking. If your pediatrician or health advisor believes your baby still needs to eat at night, make sure you keep your baby awake during the feeding, so he is still falling asleep on his own afterwards. This way, you can still teach good sleep habits, even if your baby needs to eat at night.

QUICK FIX Some babies get very sleepy during their night feeding and inevitably fall asleep. If your baby is warm, bundled, and getting his favorite thing in the world, a feeding in your arms, this is a total recipe for sleepy time. Some tricks you can try to keep your baby up include tickling his feet, burping him, uncovering or unzipping his sleep outfit, and lastly, if all else fails, you can change his diaper after the feeding.

If at any point during the sleep training you believe your baby is hungry, sick, or uncomfortable, the sleep training rules go out the window—tend to your baby. Your baby may have visible symptoms like coughing, congestion, vomiting, or fever, or he may have none at all but your parenting gut tells you that something isn't right. Those are all valid reasons to pause the sleep training and give your doc a call to schedule a checkup before resuming.

STEP 5:

repeat

NICE WORK! You've made it through the first night. Realistically, though, it will almost certainly take more than one night to see results from sleep training. I have seen results after one night, but that's pretty rare. What you are basically doing with sleep training is breaking a formed habit, whether it's rocking to sleep, feeding to sleep, or driving your baby around until she falls asleep. Along with breaking that habit, you are establishing a brand-new routine. You want to give your baby some time to do this. It wouldn't be realistic to break this habit overnight. However, if you stay consistent and repeat this plan each night for seven days, you should start seeing some good progress within a few nights.

give it a week

On average, sleep training takes about seven days to see improvement, with really good progress somewhere around nights three to five.

How fast you see progress depends on many different factors: your baby's personality, whether he is easygoing or strong-willed, how hard the crying is, if you have to take breaks during the training, your baby's age, and how long he has been used to his current routine.

Somewhere around the seven-day mark, you should notice that your baby is sleeping much better. The crying should be very minimal, if there's any at all. Your baby should be sleeping through the night or very close to it. If your baby still needs to eat, she should go right back to sleep easily after the feeding. Don't be discouraged if this is not the case; again, personality and other factors play a major role in the speed of this transition, and your baby may just need more time.

Most babies start off with about 10 hours of night sleep—this is the minimum amount of night sleep that most babies need. Once a baby starts sleeping through the night, it's the best sleep their body has ever had. It's restful and consolidated. Naturally sleeping longer than 10 hours can be difficult, but if your baby needs more sleep, she will start sleeping a little bit longer over the course of the next few weeks as her body adjusts to all of this great sleep.

Your baby may not like the routine or bedtime during the first couple of weeks. This is normal, since you are changing your baby's entire routine. Your baby may be ambivalent about all of this, or just plain furious. She may cry when you approach the bedroom or crib to let you know how unhappy she is with the new changes. It really should just be a matter of time until she adjusts, though, and starts to like her new routine. Most babies actually really enjoy their routine and going to bed after sleep training, because falling asleep is now much easier for them. It is only when they don't know how to fall asleep on their own (and know that transitioning from awake to asleep is so difficult for them) that they cry at the first sign of bedtime. Give your baby some time to adjust. My baby, who absolutely hated going to bed because she was so dependent on me, ended up being a baby who reminded ME when it was time for bed, by grabbing her lovey and pointing to her room. Many of my clients have reported similar reactions.

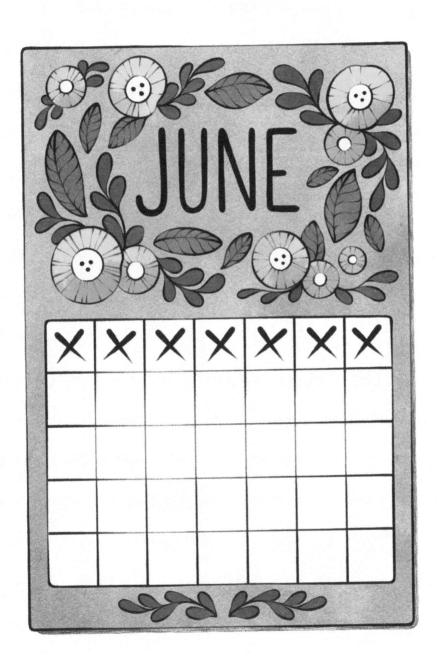

beware the peak of sleep training

There is a "peak" in sleep training, and it typically happens somewhere in the middle of the process, around night three to five. This peak occurs when a baby will cry louder and harder than any other night as a last-ditch effort for you to revert to the old routine. This can be quite frustrating, but if you know in advance that it's coming, it's easier to stay strong! The good news is that after this peak, she will usually sleep significantly better, and likely will start sleeping through the night the following night. Luckily, the peak usually only lasts one night; at most, two nights.

try again

You may have had a really tough sleep training week, or maybe you didn't even make it the full week. That's fine. Perhaps right now is not the best time. If your baby is crying too much for your liking, and comforting your baby isn't working, just take a break. Try again in a couple of weeks. You still laid a foundation this week; just pick it back up at a later date, and you may have a better outcome.

You may also want to make some changes to the plan to make it easier on both you and your baby. Perhaps you only want to work on bedtime for starters, then once you see improvement, you can move on to the first waking of the night. Or maybe you just want to work on that dreaded early morning waking (before she's gotten a solid 10 hours of sleep); perhaps try the sleep training at that time. Sure, modifying the plan may mean that it takes some more time to see progress, but you may find that this is a better alternative for you and your family. When a baby is so used to going to sleep with a sleep prop and waking at night, it is undeniably difficult to change that without either taking some time or allowing the baby to protest a bit. There isn't a sleep training method, technique, plan, book, or program on this planet that doesn't use one of these two things as its core principle.

enjoy some rest

You did it, you survived sleep training! Your baby is now sleeping better, protesting less, and falling asleep on his own, or has reached whatever goal you have set for him. Although your baby can't talk, he thanks you for how well rested he is during the day. This good rest has so many benefits, which you'll see as he's playing, giggling, and practicing his milestones. Some of the best testimonials I receive from clients are the ones reporting that their baby rolled over for the first time or took their first steps as a result of a full night's rest. Making sure a baby gets adequate sleep is so incredibly essential for growth and development, and achieving that through sleep training is so very rewarding. Great job!

sleep training faq

Q: WHY DOES MY BABY WAKE UP AS SOON AS I PUT HIM DOWN?
A: Your baby wakes up because he is likely in a very light stage of sleep. He then becomes alarmed when you lay him down, as soon as he realizes he is no longer in your arms. Ideally, this is why you want to lay your baby down completely awake, so he can fall asleep on his own.

Q: WHAT IF MY BABY CRIES THE MOMENT I LAY HER DOWN?
A: Give her a few minutes—you may be pleasantly surprised that she settles when you walk away and just give her some time to figure it out. If your baby is young, or you don't wish to leave her when she is crying, try some comforting while she remains in the crib. Once

you pick her up, it may be very difficult to lay her back down without major tears, so give the comforting in the crib a really good effort. Try some gentle noise and touch; distraction is often key.

Q: WHAT DO I DO IF MY BABY DOESN'T FALL ASLEEP?

A: Parents often fear that their baby will not fall asleep during sleep training. I can say that I have never heard of this happening, though it's a common question. Your baby will fall asleep, on average within 60 to 90 minutes on the first night. It is important to make sure that your baby's sleep schedule is appropriate so that she can fall asleep. For example, if your baby took a nap at 7:00 p.m., then she may not fall asleep for quite some time if laid down for bed at 8:00 p.m. It's also important to make sure baby is comfortably dressed and has a clean diaper.

Q: WHAT IF MY BABY DOESN'T STOP CRYING?

A: If your baby is not being comforted in any way, or is crying too much for your liking, you can first try taking him out of the room and taking a small break. Meanwhile, you can check to make sure his diaper is dry. Once he calms, try the sleep training again. If the crying continues or you feel it is excessive, you can put your baby to sleep the "old" way, then try again at the next waking.

Q: WHAT IF MY BABY THROWS UP?

A: Babies have a sensitive gag reflex, so crying can stimulate this gag reflex and cause your baby to upchuck what he just ate. Parents often think that vomiting during sleep training is caused by baby being so upset. In my experience, a baby typically throws up because they ate way too close to bedtime, and that weak gag reflex caused everything to come back up. If your baby is prone to vomiting, make sure that his last feeding is given at least 30 to 45 minutes prior to bedtime. When your baby throws up, of course change and comfort your baby. You can either resume the sleep training at the next waking or the next night. If you are concerned there's more to the vomiting than just the crying, give your pediatrician a call.

Q: WHAT IF MY BABY IS HUNGRY?

A: If you believe your baby is hungry, then by all means feed her! It's that simple. Just make sure your baby stays awake during the feeding so she can fall asleep on her own afterwards. You can do this by uncovering or unzipping your baby, tickling her feet, and discontinuing the feeding if she isn't swallowing. But if she does happen to fall asleep, just change her diaper, which will help rouse her a bit so she knows that she is going back down on her own in her own sleep space.

Q: HOW DO I KNOW IF MY BABY IS AWAKE FOR THE DAY OR IF I SHOULD PUT HIM BACK DOWN?

A: If it has been at least 10 hours from the initial bedtime, chances are your baby is awake for the day. If it is earlier than 6:00 a.m., then try giving your baby some time first, just to see if he's going to fall back asleep. If it is clear that your baby is awake and ready for the day, well, it looks like you're getting him up and starting your day, too!

Q: WHAT IF SLEEP TRAINING IS TOO STRESSFUL?

A: If sleep training is stressing you out, STOP! This should be an experience that you are positive about and confident in. You should feel good knowing that you are doing what's best for your baby. If it's anything less than that, this will not work, as it will be difficult for you to follow through. That's fine; perhaps now is just not the right time. When it is, you'll have all of the tools you need to be successful.

after the seven days

You have given your child a priceless gift—the foundation for a lifetime of good sleep habits! Now that you and your precious little one have gotten through the tough part, let's talk about some of the things you can do to ensure your baby's good sleep habits continue into the future, and what to do if any setbacks arise.

1 manage props

2 end nighttime snacktime

3 tackle naptime

4 adapt to changing schedules

5 conquer setbacks

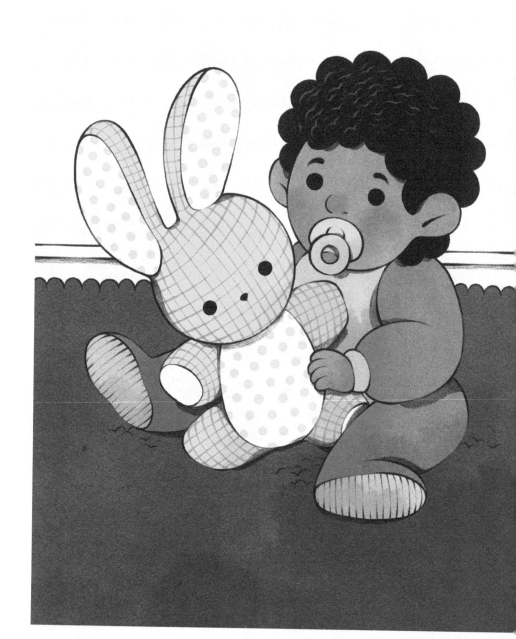

STEP 1:

manage props

HOW WE GO from an awake state to being asleep is an intricate process that involves more than just the flip of the light switch. We've talked about sleep props like rocking, swinging, mobiles, and car rides, without which your baby may be awake all night if she needs them for comfort, but there are props that can actually be helpful.

We all benefit from that something that helps us settle to sleep, whether it's a favorite blanket, the way we hold our pillow, or a certain sleep position that lulls us to sleep. All humans, whether babies or adults, wake several times a night. It's a normal part of sleep. We then use these exact same props during the night to help us get back to sleep, many times without even realizing it. It's when we don't realize we are even using a sleep prop that it can be classified as a "good" sleep prop, because it helps us back to sleep in between sleep cycles without disturbing us.

A good sleep prop for a baby can be as simple as the texture of the crib sheets or a favorite blanket. Let's talk about the two most common good sleep props—pacifiers and loveys—and how to manage them so they don't become problematic.

find binky balance

Babies are born with the innate ability to suck, so a "binky" or pacifier can be a really useful sleep prop. It helps a baby calm and settle to sleep. The best part is that somewhere between five to seven months of age, your baby will be able to pick up his own binky, usually quickly, effortlessly, and without any disruption to sleep. This is why I consider it a good sleep prop.

There is a tricky period when your baby is young and can't yet replace the binky himself. However, it's a short period, and for those first few months you'll likely still be feeding your baby during the night, so the pacifier can just be replaced after a feeding. It becomes difficult when your baby no longer needs night feedings or can go a long stretch without one, but is waking asking for a pacifier that he can't get himself. In this situation, you don't want to keep replacing the pacifier: instead, try to comfort him or go in at intervals as we discussed in the seven-day plan. He can still have the pacifier when he goes to sleep, but if it falls out, it's best to help him learn to settle in other ways.

If your baby continues to wake and be disrupted by the pacifier, then that prop may need to be eliminated completely. In this case, you would just take away the pacifier and settle him in other ways until he forgets about the pacifier and no longer cries for it. This transition typically takes somewhere from a few nights up to a week.

try a lovey

A "lovey," or security object, can be a powerful tool for settling a baby to sleep and helping ease those natural night wakings. During the first 12 months, however, it's not recommended that a baby sleep with anything in his crib—not even a blanket. So for the first year you can use the lovey to help settle, calm, and prepare your baby for sleep, but don't leave it with him, because it's a SIDS risk factor.

EXTRA HELP: SAYING GOODBYE TO BINKY

If your baby uses a binky, there is another time when it will get tricky again. That's when your baby becomes a toddler, and it's time to say bye-bye to the binky for good. Most pediatricians and dentists recommend eliminating the pacifier by two years of age to prevent oral and dental problems. This can be stressful for parents and toddlers, but there are many fun ways to do it. Here are a couple:

- **BINKY FAIRY.** You can tell your child that it's time for the binky fairy to come and take her pacifiers to give them to babies who need them. In exchange, she will leave a thank-you note and a gift.

- **GARBAGE CAN.** This may sound silly, but for younger children, the only way they may understand that something is gone forever is if it goes in the garbage can. Most kids, even at a young age, understand that once something goes in the garbage, it doesn't come back out. So explain ahead of time that it's time to say goodbye to the binky. Have him place all the pacifiers in there, and that's it! You can give your child a gift in return for his bravery.

- **BUILD-A-BEAR.** Bring your child to a Build-A-Bear Workshop, have her pick out a favorite teddy, and put the binky inside when they stuff it. Now your child still has her beloved binky *and* a new buddy to sleep with! You can also easily do this with any teddy if you or a friend knows how to sew.

There's a wide range of common loveys that babies use for comfort, including stuffed animals, Mom's T-shirt, a receiving blanket, or even the silky tags on a bib or an article of clothing, to name a few. Babies come to associate the textures, colors, and scents of these transitional objects with snuggles and cozy time.

Some babies get attached to a lovey very easily, while others show no interest at all. Here are some tips to help your baby accept a lovey:

OFFER A LOVEY WHILE YOUR BABY IS FEEDING. This is how most babies start to get attached to a lovey. The feeding is comforting, and holding a security object during this time helps build an attachment to it. After some time, your baby should start to connect the dots that the lovey offers comfort and security. If your baby is too young to hold a lovey, just put it up against his cheek as he is eating as a way of introducing and facilitating the attachment to a security object.

FOLLOW YOUR BABY'S LEAD. Look for clues and signs that your baby is interested in an object. Does he show particular interest in a certain teddy? Does he calm when he plays with his bib? Is he often searching for the same toy? These are all great clues that your baby is drawn to something—and the start of a beautiful relationship with their lovey.

DON'T FORCE IT. If your baby isn't interested in a lovey, don't force it. Some babies either need time or aren't interested in any other comfort than just being in your arms.

end nighttime snacktime

MANY EXPERTS AGREE that somewhere between the age of three and six months, most healthy babies are capable of sleeping through the night without needing to eat. When your baby reaches a point in her development when she no longer *needs* the feedings for nutrition, she may still continue to wake and *want* the feedings for comfort. There's no way to know with 100 percent certainty if your baby is waking for hunger or for comfort. However, there are two clues to consider:

» If your baby is just suckling and not audibly swallowing, she may be comfort sucking.

» If she starts to drift off as soon as you give her the feeding, or isn't really interested in eating, this too may be a sign that she just wants to comfort feed.

On the flip side, some babies who aren't really that hungry will nurse or down a bottle just because it's offered—just as you might eat your very favorite food if someone put it in front of your face, even if you weren't hungry!

If you're unsure, the best thing to do is speak with your pediatrician about whether or not your baby still needs to eat at night. Age, weight, growth patterns, and development are often our strongest and most reliable indicators as to whether a baby is eating because he is hungry or just because he wants to be comforted to sleep. Once your pediatrician has given you the green light to eliminate night feedings, you can do so in one of several ways.

go cold turkey

This method is the most firm, and again, for several reasons, you'll want to make sure that your pediatrician is okay with abrupt elimination of feedings. The doctor can confirm that your baby no longer needs feedings. If cold turkey is acceptable to your doctor, you can respond to wakings with verbal or comfort check-ins.

If your baby has only been comfort suckling and not really eating much, this may work well. The cold turkey method sends the clear message that baby will no longer be receiving comfort feedings. Your baby may be initially quite upset, but a clear message yields much faster progress, and in the end, less crying, since sleep improves quickly. If your baby is used to getting several pretty large night feedings, though, you may not want to abruptly cut him off. In those cases, weaning would be more appropriate.

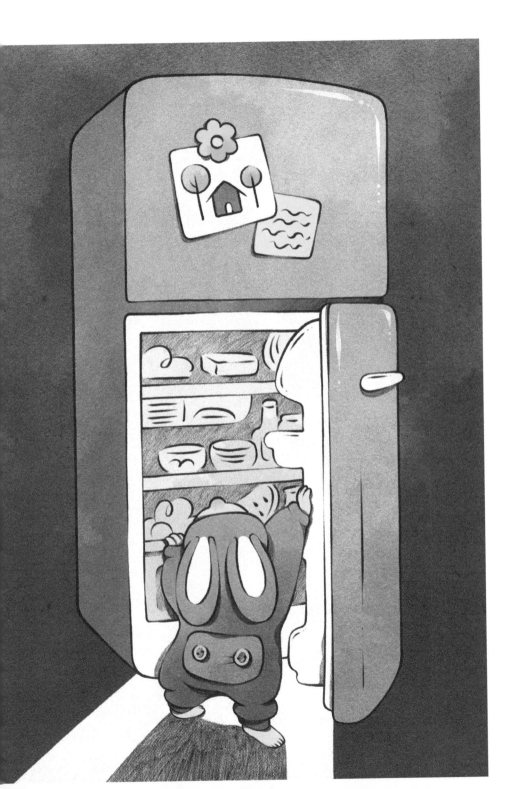

wean or decrease feedings

You can wean your baby from night feedings by decreasing the amount you offer at each waking. If your baby is getting, say, 4 ounces two times a night, you can start by cutting back to 3 ounces two times a night. In a couple of nights, decrease to 2 ounces at each feeding, and so forth. If you're breastfeeding, simply decrease the time you breastfeed, since you won't know the exact amount. Either way, this should be a gradual decrease.

This chart shows an example of a weaning schedule for a baby who is eating 6 ounces of formula at night or breastfeeding for 20 minutes:

	AMOUNT OF FORMULA	TIME BREASTFEEDING
NIGHT 1	5 ounces	15 minutes
NIGHT 2	4 ounces	12 minutes
NIGHT 3	3 ounces	10 minutes
NIGHT 4	2 ounces	8 minutes
NIGHT 5	1 ounce	5 minutes
NIGHT 6	.5 ounce	2 minutes
NIGHT 7	No more feeding	No more feeding

This is just a sample outline. Please speak with your pediatrician before trying to night wean.

use a mixed approach

You can also use a combination of methods, such as cold turkey for the comfort feeding wakings that occur very early in the night, then the weaning method for the wakings that occur after a long stretch of sleep.

So let's say, for example, that your baby wakes at 10:00 p.m. every night, but you know he can't possibly be hungry, since you just fed him at bedtime. Here you would just provide verbal or comfort check-ins until your baby falls back asleep. Then if baby wakes again at, say, 2:00 a.m., you would give a smaller feeding as part of the weaning plan.

trade one prop for another

Another way to eliminate comfort feedings is by replacing them with another form of comfort. Comfort feedings are a powerful sleep prop, and by far the most difficult prop to eliminate. If you can get your baby to accept some rocking or holding instead, they will be much easier to eliminate. When a baby is reliant on comfort feedings, other props are not as desirable, but they can offer a good distraction.

QUICK FIX Since comfort feedings usually come at night, you'll want to keep the substitute props short, simple, and not too stimulating. These can include rocking, holding, or even just shushing.

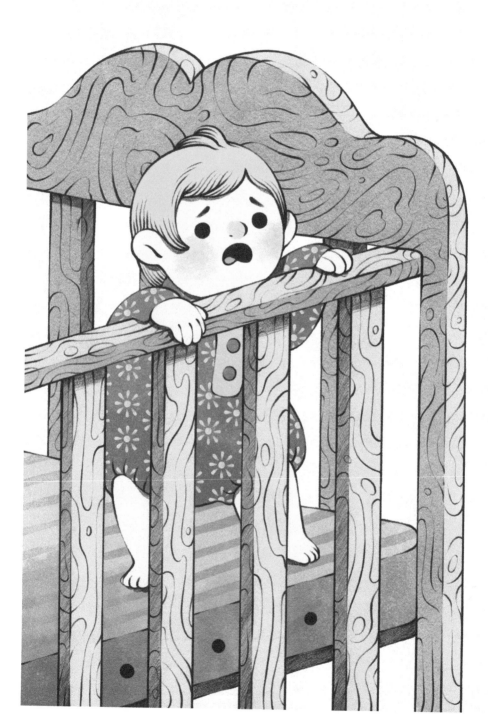

tackle naptime

SOMETIMES NAPS IMPROVE on their own over time, but some nap training is often necessary. Consistency in the overall sleep routine is important, so handling naps in a similar way to nighttime will improve your baby's sleep routine more quickly. Here are some tips to assist in nap training.

set a schedule

Putting your baby down to sleep at the right time is important, especially when she is still taking more than two daily naps. At this point, use your baby's sleepy cues, as opposed to a clock-based schedule, to decide on the right waking period in between sleep times. The trick is to find the perfect middle ground: not to put your baby down too tired, but tired enough that she can fall asleep easily.

Once your baby is down to a two-nap schedule, or her naps are pretty consistent, putting her down at about the same time each day will work well. Her internal clock will help her settle to sleep at those times if you generally keep them consistent.

Here are some typical nap schedules at different ages:

AGE	NAPTIMES	BEDTIME
3 to 4 months	1.5 to 2 hours of awake time between naps	8:00 to 8:30 p.m.
6 to 7 months	2.5 hours of awake time between naps	6:30 to 7:00 p.m. if 2 naps 7:00 to 8:30 p.m. if 3 naps
8 to 10 months	9:00 or 10:00 a.m. nap 1 2:00 p.m. nap 2	7:00 to 8:00 p.m.
12 to 18 months	10:00 a.m. and 2:00 p.m. if 2 naps 11:30 a.m. or 12:00 p.m. if 1 nap	8:00 to 8:30 p.m. if 2 naps 7:00 to 7:30 p.m. if 1 nap

use your routine

A naptime routine is as important as a bedtime routine, just a little shorter. It helps cue your baby that sleep time is coming and keeps things consistent. This routine should also be simple enough to be portable, so you can easily implement it when you are on the go. An easy naptime routine might include a diaper change, snuggles, a key phrase like "it's sleepy time," and putting your baby down to sleep.

put baby down awake

Naps can be quite difficult for a baby to master, sometimes with many tears involved—but you can do so much to help! We've talked about how putting your baby down awake at sleep times is important so when your baby transitions between sleep cycles, he can do that without needing any assistance from you. The same is true of daytime nap cycles. It can be very difficult for a baby to fall back asleep after waking during the day—this is typically why some babies only catnap.

Similar to night training, nap training involves the following steps:

1. After your naptime routine, put your baby down in his crib awake.

2. Go in at intervals to comfort or reassure your baby (page 51).

3. If your baby doesn't fall asleep in an hour's time, take him out of the room, take a break for 20 or 25 minutes, then try again.

4. If your baby is crying the entire time and just having a horrible time falling asleep, then you may even need to take him out sooner—perhaps the timing just wasn't right. Sometimes taking a break, resetting, and trying again at a different time results in a much better outcome.

QUICK FIX During naptime, resist the urge to run in at the first squeak. Keep in mind that sometimes babies make noise in between sleep cycles or while they sleep, and it takes a baby a few minutes to really wake up. Left alone, your baby may fall back asleep, resulting in a longer nap than just a catnap.

Overall, use your best judgment—you're the parent and you know your baby best! If you follow your baby's lead and don't force the issue, you will get into a groove.

naptime faq

Q: WHAT SHOULD I DO IF MY BABY HAS MISSED A NAP?

A: If you are out and about, or have lost track of time, and your baby misses his nap, just put him down as soon as you can. If it is late in the day, I'd recommend just giving him a short catnap so the nap doesn't interfere with bedtime. If it's the last nap of the day, you can also just put him down for bed earlier.

Q: WHAT IF MY BABY REFUSES TO NAP?

A: If your baby is refusing a nap but is absolutely tired and needs one, you can try taking a stroller walk, walking her around in a baby carrier, or putting her into a swing or anywhere else where she'll get sleepy and can be safely supervised. I wouldn't do this regularly while you are sleep training, but you can certainly use this as backup. If it's late in the day, you can wake her up after a short catnap so as not to interfere with bedtime, or you can skip the nap completely and just put your baby down early for the night.

Q: WHAT IF MY BABY ONLY CATNAPS?

A: It is not unusual for a baby who is reliant on sleep props to only catnap. If he's using a prop to get to sleep, he will likely wake after one sleep cycle (30 to 45 minutes) and expect that prop. This results in a cycle of persistent catnapping. Once your baby learns to fall asleep on his own, these catnaps will resolve. To help aid this process, give your waking baby a few minutes to see if he will fall back asleep. Taking him out of the crib right away may reinforce the catnapping, as leaving the crib sends him the message that, "okay, naptime's over."

Q: WHAT IF I NEED TO GO OUT DURING NAPTIME?

A: Parents often worry that they have to be home for every naptime. You could drive yourself crazy with this! The truth is, you don't always need to be home. An occasional car seat or stroller nap is fine. You will not wreck your baby's sleep habits because you wanted to go to the park for the day and she fell asleep on the way home. If your baby is going to be napping while you're out, try to let her nap at her regular naptime—just don't allow naps that are much longer than they usually are, as this can interfere with night sleep. Other than that, go out, have fun, and enjoy your baby during outings!

Q: WHAT DO I DO IF MY BABY FELL ASLEEP DURING THE CAR RIDE HOME WHEN I WASN'T PLANNING IT?

A: Just let your baby finish her nap. You can take the long way home to at least get a catnap in, or quietly sneak her car seat into a dim room when you get home, and stay with her. Don't attempt to take her out of the car seat and transfer her into the crib: 99 percent of the time my clients do this, their baby wakes right up. The only time transferring to the crib works is at bedtime, when sleep is much deeper. Again, remember safety first: Make sure your baby is supervised, or transferred into a crib if you feel she is in an unsafe sleep position—even if that ends the nap.

Q: MY BABY HATES THE CAR SEAT, AND CRIES HYSTERICALLY THE WHOLE TIME HE'S IN IT! IS THIS TYPICAL?

A: It is very common for a baby, in particular one who does not know how to sleep independently, to hate the car seat. He knows that settling to sleep is very difficult for him without props, and he views the car seat as a "no prop zone." In other words, he knows that during the time he is in a car seat, Mom or Dad can't feed or hold him to sleep. Babies who are dependent on props that require a parent's help typically dislike the car seat until they learn to sleep independently. Once independent sleep is mastered, your baby will love the car seat, and maybe a little bit too much!

Q: DOES THE ROOM HAVE TO BE DARK DURING NAPTIME?

A: Ideally during sleep training, I recommend that the room be as dark as you can get it. Light can make it difficult for a baby to fall asleep, and sleeping during the day is already hard enough—after all, they're missing the action! If there's any way you can make this process go more smoothly, like making the room dark, I say go for it.

Q: I WORRY THAT IF I ALWAYS MAKE THE ROOM DARK, MY BABY WILL NOT NAP IN OTHER CIRCUMSTANCES. ANY ADVICE?

A: A dark environment promotes sleep, but once a baby's sleep pressure (her need for sleep) increases, there's no way of stopping sleep. Your baby will sleep when she gets tired enough. Oh, she may struggle a little more or take her nap later than usual if it's light and she's used to dark, but be assured, she will nap. The struggle is not necessarily related to being used to sleeping in a dark room at home. Even babies who don't typically sleep in a dark environment may struggle with naps in daylight or bright rooms, simply because light suppresses melatonin, the hormone that promotes sleep.

Q: DOES MY BABY HAVE TO WEAR PAJAMAS OR A SLEEP SACK AT NAPTIME?

A: You don't have to change your baby into pajamas at naptime, as long as he has comfy clothes on without any bumps, zippers, big buttons, or anything that would make your little one uncomfortable. A sleep sack can be helpful, since it acts as a blanket but is safe. It offers warmth and comfort, and some babies use it for soothing. It's also safe to use when a baby rolls because it does not interfere with rolling, and is loose enough on the leg area to allow movement in any direction baby wants.

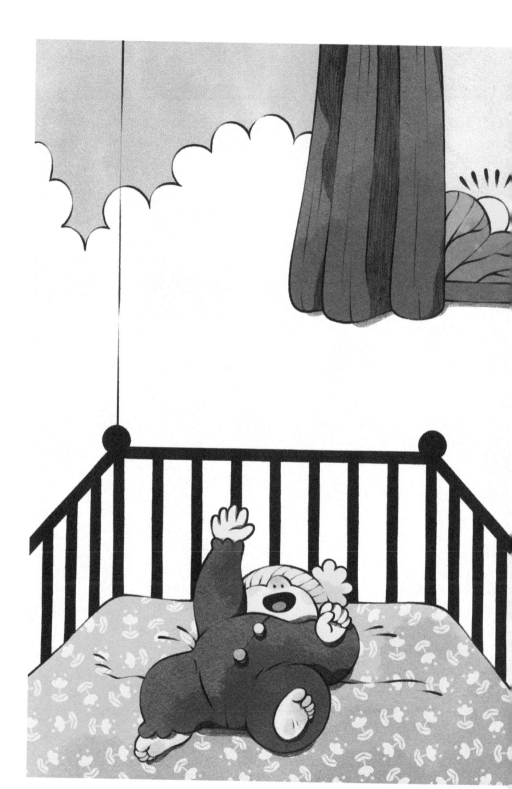

adapt to changing schedules

AS BABIES GROW their sleep needs evolve, which often means dropping a nap or moving bedtime or wake-up time. Just when you have everything running smoothly, these changes can shake things up a bit. Never fear, though: With the strategies below, you'll weather these transitions easily.

help baby drop a nap

Once your baby has mastered independent sleep at naptimes, daytime sleep should be a breeze . . . until it's time to drop a nap! Nap transitions can make things go haywire again, but luckily it's an easy fix that just requires a shift in the schedule.

Here are some signs that your baby is ready to drop a nap:

» Your baby is taking more time to fall asleep at naptimes. This is a clue that your baby's awake period in between sleep times needs to be increased—which often results in one less nap.

» Your baby's naps are getting shorter and shorter. This typically affects the last nap of the day, but sometimes it can impact other naps.

» Your baby is fighting naptime and sometimes completely refuses to nap.

» Your baby's last nap of the day is starting to interfere with bedtime.

This chart shows the average ages for nap transitions:

AGE	NUMBER OF NAPS
0 to 2 months	Several naps
3 to 4 months	4 naps
4 to 5 months	Transition to 3 naps
6 to 8 months	Transition to 2 naps
10 to 18 months	Transition to 1 nap
22 months to 3.5 years	Drop final nap

For some babies, nap transitions are as clear as day: She fights her naps and takes a long time to fall asleep at naptimes. Other babies fall asleep just fine at naptimes, but have a hard time at bedtime, and some even start waking at night. In those cases, it's not as obvious that the sleep troubles are directly related to a nap transition—at first, you might not realize the cause. My best advice is that when you suspect a nap transition is underway, just try dropping a nap. Look at the chart: If your baby is around an age when a nap transition typically occurs, and she's showing some signs, give it a go! If it turns out that this wasn't the best choice after all, you can always go back and try again in a few weeks when your baby may be more ready.

Here's how to drop a nap smoothly:

INCREASE AWAKE PERIODS. This may happen naturally. Some babies start staying awake longer in between sleep times, and this prompts the nap transition. If this has not happened naturally, try to increase your baby's awake periods by at least 20 or 30 minutes to accommodate the new schedule. Without doing this, you'll end up with a really long awake period in the evening before bedtime, which can cause a new host of issues.

TRY AN EARLIER BEDTIME. Dropping a nap will typically result in an earlier bedtime until your baby starts to tolerate longer awake periods. Since you can only increase those awake periods so much before she gets cranky and overtired, an earlier bedtime is almost inevitable during nap transitions. When shifting baby's bedtime, however, you don't want to make an abrupt change since her internal clock may already be set to go to sleep at a certain time. Try a 20- or 30-minute shift for a few nights before making any further changes, then continue the shift gradually.

GIVE IT A WEEK. Anytime you make a change in your baby's schedule, it will take about a week for his internal clock to reset. Give it at least a week before you decide if dropping a nap was the right choice. If there was an improvement in your baby's sleep, then you know you did the right thing. If his sleep worsened, then he may need a few more weeks before you drop the nap.

ACCEPT EVENING CRANKINESS. Crankiness during the evening hours is not an indication that a nap transition is not successful. As the evening approaches, your baby's sleep pressure increases. Sleep pressure, or the need for sleep, is naturally lowest in the morning after a good night's rest. As the day goes on, the pressure accumulates, and naps don't completely relieve this pressure. By the evening, sleep pressure is high. Can't you relate? We adults are often at our most tired and cranky at the end of the day, too! It is only a good night's sleep that resets this sleep pressure. So as long as your baby is sleeping well and is generally happy, some crankiness as the day wears on is normal.

move bedtime or wake-up time

An ideal bedtime for a baby is between 7:00 and 8:30 p.m., and a good wake-up time falls between 6:00 and 8:30 a.m. If bedtime is too early or too late, this can cause sleep troubles. Wake-up time is usually determined by how many hours a baby can sleep at night. If you feel that your baby's bedtime schedule needs adjusting, here are some ways to shift bedtime and wake-up time:

» Shift the entire schedule by 15 minutes each day until you reach the desired bedtime/wake-up time.

» Give it at least a week. Changing a baby's internal clock can take about that long.

» Keep in mind, many babies only need 10 hours of nighttime sleep. So if your baby goes to bed at 7:00 p.m., 5:00 a.m. may be a normal time for her to be awake (even if you're not ready to get up!). In this case, I wouldn't try to force more sleep if she looks well rested; instead, shift her bedtime to a later one. Again, you can do this by making 15-minute shifts each night.

EXTRA HELP: DAYLIGHT SAVING TIME

The aforementioned strategies also work when adjusting a baby's schedule for daylight saving time. That one hour can throw things off kilter; after all, the clock may have changed, but your baby did not get the memo! To smooth the daylight saving transition, you may wish to start a week before daylight saving time so you can ease into the new schedule. It's also helpful to use blackout blinds—and be sure to use your relaxing bedtime routine so baby knows, "yes, it's really sleepy time."

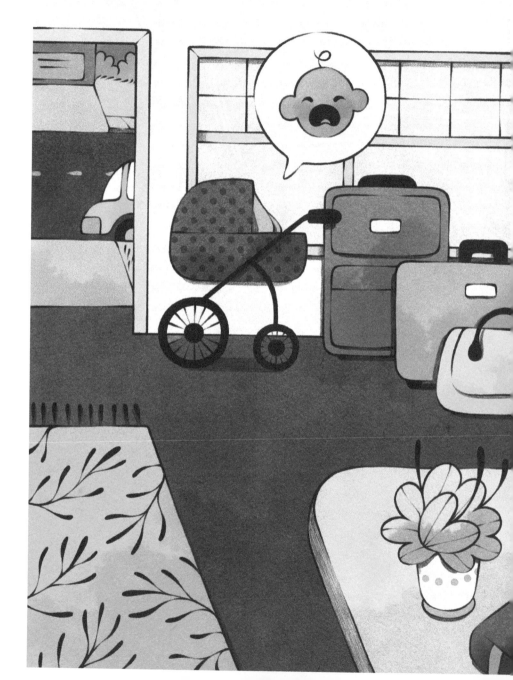

conquer setbacks

BABIES ARE CONSTANTLY growing and changing in profound ways. Think about all of the changes that occur in just the first 12 months of a baby's life! Your baby grows from a helpless newborn to an active toddler, from learning to adapt to life outside the womb to rolling, crawling, standing, walking, and even saying first words. There is major cognitive and physical development going on during the first year, resulting in a total transformation. This amazing growth continues into toddlerhood and beyond, and you will marvel. When you think about this growth, it's easy to understand why good sleep is important. Your baby's body is working hard to achieve all of these milestones!

By helping your baby gain good sleep habits, you are giving your baby such a gift! Once she is sleep trained, she'll sleep significantly better, and will be equipped to breeze through these developments. However, considering the speedy rate at which your baby is developing, setbacks are to be expected. There will also be times when your baby just isn't feeling well. So let's talk about these possible hiccups along the way and what you can do to keep things on track.

handle developmental leaps

We've already touched on this in the "Choose Your Moment" section, and you can refer back to the list to see when many developmental leaps occur (see page 33). That said, it is not unusual for a baby who is learning to roll over, crawl, stand, or achieve any other milestone to have a hard time settling to sleep for the night. All your baby wants to do is practice her new skills, even when it's time to sleep. She may even wake in the middle of the night and practice some more! The first few times this happens, you may think it's cute, but when your baby is in her crib partying all night and keeping everyone up, you may not be so thrilled about the situation. Here's how you can help your little one get through her developmental leaps:

PROVIDE LOTS OF PRACTICE TIME. If your baby is learning a new skill, give him lots of practice time on a mat or other area that is comfortable but firm. Babies like to practice their skills in the crib because it is a perfect surface for rolling, crawling, or standing. They can do it with ease, especially with those awesome crib slats to grab onto. Providing your baby plenty of time to do this on a proper surface during the day means he will be less likely to do it when it's time to sleep.

RESIST STARTING ANY NEW BAD SLEEP HABITS. Just because your baby is staying up late practicing a new skill does not mean you need to revert to sleep-inducing props such as rocking, holding, or feeding to sleep. This prolongs the regression, as it's preventing her from practicing these skills and figuring out a way to get to sleep in spite of these new developments.

ALLOW FOR THEIR LEARNING PROCESS. Extra comfort is okay when your baby is having a hard time learning a new skill, and you can comfort your baby as he gets frustrated or cries, but try not to interfere with the process. Jumping in to stop his cries as he is learning a new skill doesn't help or speed up the process; in fact, it can hinder it. The faster your baby learns, the faster he will return to his good sleep patterns.

travel with baby

Even if you're a seasoned traveler, traveling with a baby can be stressful. The sleep environment is not ideal, and a schedule can be difficult to maintain. This often worries parents, and some even avoid traveling altogether. I encourage you to go! Trust me when I say that a temporary situation like a vacation is not going to undo all of your hard work. In fact, the best part about sleep training a baby is that these skills stay in place—your baby will not suddenly unlearn how to sleep. In fact, you may be surprised at how well your baby sleeps in different environments, because she has her independent sleep skills in place. And hey, worst-case scenario, your baby's sleep gets a bit out of sync on vacation. It will only take a couple of nights to get back to normal when you get home. You do not have to completely re-train your baby; at most, you'll just need to remind her of the skills that she already has in place. Here's how you can stay on track as you travel:

TRY TO KEEP NORMAL SLEEP TIMES. You can help your baby fall asleep more easily and stay on track if you still put him down at his normal sleep times no matter where you are. He can nap in a car seat, stroller, or on you during a flight at his regular sleep time. He may struggle a bit because the environment is different, or he may take longer to fall asleep, but you can help by staying calm, since your baby senses your energy. Sooner or later, he will fall asleep!

BRING A TRAVEL CRIB. If you're on vacation or otherwise away from home for a few nights, plan for a separate sleep space for your baby. There's no reason to start new sleep habits that you don't intend on keeping when you get back home. Most hotels provide travel cribs, or you can bring a portable one of your own.

FOCUS ON THE FUN. Sleep may not be perfect during travel or vacation, and that's fine. You can always get right back on track when you get home. Don't stress; enjoy your trip!

GIVE JET LAG TIME TO RESOLVE. If you travel to a different time zone, your baby will likely sleep at different times than she is used to. When you get back home, she may also experience some jet lag, and will have difficulty settling to sleep at her usual times. The best advice I have for jet lag is to just give it time. It typically only takes a few nights, up to a week, for an internal clock to shift back to normal after traveling across time zones. Stick to your baby's normal home schedule and routine as much as possible, and it will fall into place.

survive teething, colds, fevers . . .

There will be times when your baby gets sick, has a fever, or is uncomfortable—this can certainly throw sleep routines out of whack. Here's how to handle these setbacks:

ILLNESS. Whenever a baby is sick, in pain, or uncomfortable, sleep training rules should go out the window. Comfort and tend to your baby—her health and wellness are your number-one priority. You can always get back on track when she is feeling better. And chances are, if she is already sleep trained, she will go right back to sleeping well on her own when she's feeling better.

VACCINATIONS. Vaccines can alter sleep. Many babies actually sleep longer after a vaccination because their body is going through an immune response, producing antibodies as if she was fighting an infection. This can be taxing on a baby's body, so they typically sleep longer than usual. However, some babies struggle with sleep after a vaccine because they are uncomfortable, either due to pain from the injection or because of a low-grade fever. Luckily, symptoms from vaccines typically only last 24 to 48 hours, and should be treated in the same way as you would an illness. Which again means sleep-training rules go out the window!

TEETHING. If you believe your baby is in pain from teething, speak with your pediatrician about proper pain control. Addressing the pain will help prevent any discomfort at bedtime or during the night. But keep in mind that just because a baby is teething—signs include chewing, biting, or drooling—it doesn't mean he is in pain. Sure, it's perhaps annoying, but it's not always painful, and usually it's not enough to wake a sleeping baby. It's also worth noting that when babies do experience pain from teething, it's typically right before and after the tooth erupts. Teething symptoms do not usually last for weeks. Many parents tell me that their baby has been waking for weeks "because he is teething." Scientifically, this is not very likely. Look for more specific pain symptoms that may occur right before the tooth erupts, like red, swollen gums that feel painful to baby when touched, and a white bud poking through.

SOMETHING IS JUST NOT RIGHT. There will be times when you just don't know what is wrong. Your baby is not settling to sleep, is crying harder than usual, looks uncomfortable, and something just isn't sitting right. Always trust that intuition and give your pediatrician a call. Your doctor can rule out any medical conditions or other issues that might be causing sleep troubles. And don't feel you need to force sleep training during these times. Good sleep will come in due time when your baby is feeling better.

QUICK FIX If you really feel like baby's sleep is being disrupted by illness, teething, or other issues, the best thing you can do for her is stay calm and address her issues. Your intuition will guide you, and when you feel like you're in uncharted territory, reach out to others for advice. Don't be intimidated about a midnight call to the doctor, or be afraid to push for what you feel like you need. You're advocating for your baby, and that's exactly what you should be doing!

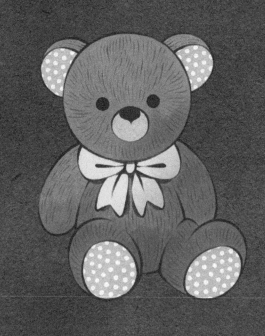

EPILOGUE

CONGRATULATIONS ON MAKING IT THIS FAR! You've made the decision to get better sleep for you, your baby, and your family, and now you are reaping the benefits.

Was it easy? Probably not. Was it worth it? Absolutely! Anything that contributes to the health and well-being of a baby (and you as a parent) is always worthwhile, in my opinion.

And it turns out that your baby doesn't hate you for this, right? He loves you for so many reasons, including the gift of sleep you have given him. He can finally be a well-rested and happy baby, and you can let go of your guilt or frustration about the bad sleep habits that were making him so miserable.

Parenting a child is momentous. It is by far one of the most important things you will ever do in your life. You are responsible for raising a human being! At times you will have to make some really tough decisions. At times you will feel such joy and happiness, and at other times immense stress and frustration. But no matter where you are on that spectrum, know that as long as you have your baby's best interests at heart, that roller coaster of emotions is just par for the course. You're doing a great job!

Now it's your turn. After you put your baby to bed, go enjoy that glass of wine or warm tea. Binge-watch your favorite shows, cuddle up with a good book, and enjoy your partner, now that your baby isn't sleeping in between you two anymore. And don't worry: Those are just phantom cries; your baby is sleeping soundly in her crib. She is sleep trained!

RESOURCES

WHEN IT COMES TO BABIES AND SLEEP, there is so much information out there on the Web. And with that, so much misinformation! My website, VioletSleepBabySleep.com, aims to simplify this by providing useful, fun, and evidence-based advice. Here are some other trustworthy websites you can count on:

BabySleep.com

NICHD.nih.gov

SleepFoundation.org

Here are a few other good books on the subjects of baby care and sleep training:

The No-Cry Sleep Solution: Gentle Ways to Help Your Baby Sleep Through the Night by Elizabeth Pantley

The Science of Mom: A Research-Based Guide to Your Baby's First Year by Alice Green Callahan

Secrets of the Baby Whisperer by Tracy Hogg and Melinda Blau

Sleeping Through the Night, Revised Edition: How Infants, Toddlers, and Their Parents Can Get a Good Night's Sleep by Jodi A. Mindell

To help with that bedtime routine, here's a list of my favorite baby bedtime books:

Big Enough for a Bed (Sesame Street) by Apple Jordan

Goodnight Moon by Margaret Wise Brown

I Love You Through and Through by Bernadette Rossetti-Shustak

Llama Llama Red Pajama by Anna Dewdney

Twinkle, Twinkle, Time for Bed by Children's Press

REFERENCES

Cohen, Gail M., and Laurie W. Albertini. "Colic." Pediatrics in Review. July 01, 2012. Accessed March 07, 2018. http://pedsinreview. aappublications.org/content/33/7/332.

Hauck, Fern R., Olanrewaju O. Omojokun, and Mir S. Siadaty. "Do Pacifiers Reduce the Risk of Sudden Infant Death Syndrome? A Meta-analysis." Pediatrics. November 01, 2005. Accessed March 07, 2018. http://pediatrics.aappublications.org/content/116/5/e716.

Hugh, Sarah C., Nikolaus E. Wolter, Evan J. Propst, Karen A. Gordon, Sharon L. Cushing, and Blake C. Papsin. "Infant Sleep Machines and Hazardous Sound Pressure Levels." Pediatrics. March 03, 2014. Accessed March 07, 2018. http://pediatrics.aappublications.org/ content/early/2014/02/25/peds.2013-3617

International Hip Dysplasia Institute. "Hip-Healthy Swaddling." Accessed March 07, 2018. https://hipdysplasia.org/ developmental-dysplasia-of-the-hip/hip-healthy-swaddling

National Sleep Foundation. "What Happens When You Sleep?" Accessed March 07, 2018. https://sleepfoundation.org /how-sleep-works/what-happens-when-you-sleep.

Niemelä, M., O. Pihakari, T. Pokka, and M. Uhari. "Pacifier as a Risk Factor for Acute Otitis Media: A Randomized, Controlled Trial of Parental Counseling." Advances in Pediatrics. September 2000. Accessed March 07, 2018. https://www.ncbi.nlm.nih.gov /pubmed/10969091.

Williamson, A. M. "Moderate Sleep Deprivation Produces Impairments in Cognitive and Motor Performance Equivalent to Legally Prescribed Levels of Alcohol Intoxication." Occupational and Environmental Medicine 57, no. 10 (2000): 649-55. doi:10.1136 /oem.57.10.649.

INDEX

A

awake-time
  awake period,
    increasing, 94, 95
  feedings, keeping baby awake
    during, 63, 71
  full awakening, time needed
    for, 62
  noise during the day, 5
  sample schedules, 22, 86
  wake-up time, adjusting, 96
awake-to-sleep training
  excessive crying during
    attempts, 55, 58
  falling asleep alone as
    goal, 47, 69
  first night
    misconceptions, 40
  flow chart, 53
  as last step of bedtime
    routine, 48–49
  naptime concerns, 87
  newborns, practice with, 10

B

baby cameras, 54
bath time, keeping separate, 26
bed sharing, avoiding, 15
bedtime
  bedtime routines, 22, 26, 48, 49
  catnaps, not interfering with
    bedtime, 88
  consistent bedtime,
    importance of, 24
  crying at first sign of
    bedtime, 66
  dim room as helpful, 5
  early bedtimes, 95
  ideal bedtime, 25, 96
  last feeding before bedtime,
    timing of, 70
  last nap before bedtime,
    dropping, 94
  for newborns, 10–11, 25
  refusal of bedtime as
    a test, 35
  skills, wanting to practice at
    bedtime, 34

staying out past bedtime, 27

teething discomfort and, 103

transfer from car seat to crib
at bedtime, 89

binkies, 76, 77

blankets

cribs, keeping blankets out
of, 8, 14, 76

receiving blankets as
loveys, 77

removal of, when
co-sleeping, 15

as sleep props, 75

sleep sacks as an
alternative, 91

swaddles as preferable, 6

breaks

from colicky babies, 8

from crying babies, 68, 70

from newborns, 7

during sleep training,
41, 58, 65, 87

Build-A-Bear, 77

C

car seats, 89–90, 101

catnapping, 5, 22, 87, 88, 89

check-ins, 51–55, 80, 83

colic, 8

comfort check-ins

cold turkey, checking in
when totally eliminating
feedings, 80

crib, comforting baby in, 69

flow chart example, 53

illness, comforting during,
70, 102

intervals, deciding
upon, 51–52

laying baby down awake, 87

for newborns, 3, 10

pacifier use, early days, 76

skill learning and
milestones, extra comfort
during, 32, 100

verbal check-ins, 54

comfort feedings, 79, 80, 83

co-sleeping, 15

crankiness, 30, 95, 96

cribs

bare cribs as ideal, 8, 76

car seat-to-crib
transfer, 89–90

catnaps and, 88

comforting babies in, 69

crib bumpers, avoiding, 14

laying baby down
awake, 48, 53, 87

as safest sleep space, 9

skills practiced in, 100

tips for getting used to
crib, 18–19

travel cribs, 101

crying

check-ins and, 55

colicky babies, soothing, 8

crying (*continued*)
  cribs, crying when laid
    down in, 18
  decrease in crying with
    routine acceptance, 38
  naptime, cutting short due to
    crying, 87
  of newborns, 5–6
  sleep training, crying
    due to, 33, 42–43, 58
  verbal check-ins, crying
    diminishing with, 54
  waiting intervals, 52

D

dark sleep environment,
  maintaining, 15, 90
daylight saving time, 97
day-night confusion, 4–5, 33
daytime noise, 5, 16
daytime sleep, 5, 87, 93
drowsy signs, 23

F

feedings
  bedtime routine, as
    part of, 48
  comfort feedings, 79, 80, 83
  crib time, trying after
    feedings, 19
  daytime feedings, making a
    priority, 5, 11
  feeding-to-sleep, 22, 23, 30,
    40–41, 55, 100

loveys, introducing during
  feedings, 78
of newborns, 4, 10, 33
night feedings, 31, 42,
  63–64, 66, 76, 80
past bedtime, 27
staying awake during, 71
vomiting after feedings, 70
weaning schedule, 82

G

goal setting, 19, 38, 40, 59
growth spurts, 33, 34

H

hats, not needed for sleep, 18

I

illness, refraining from sleep
  training during, 32, 64, 102

J

jet lag, 102

K

key phrase use, 27, 49, 51,
  53, 54, 86

L

loveys, 66, 76–78
lullabies, use in bedtime
  routines, 5, 10, 26

M

melatonin as a sleep
  promoter, 4, 15, 33, 90
mobiles, 16, 18

N

naptime
  apparel choices, 91
  awake, laying baby down
    when, 87
  car-ride napping, 89–90
  dark sleep
    environment, 15, 90
  dropping a nap, 93–95
  missing naps, 88
  napping in parent's arms, 9
  for newborns, 5, 12
  sample nap schedules,
    22, 24, 85–86
newborns
  bedtime routine, 10, 26
  crying of, 5–6, 8
  hats, avoiding use of, 18
  naps, 5, 12, 24
  Rock 'N Play, use of, 9
  sleep cycles as erratic, 3–4
  tips on settling
    newborns, 6–7
  witching hour, 10, 25
night wakings
  assisting baby to sleep
    leading to, 48
  family discussions on, 41
  intervention, delaying, 61–62
  key phrase, repeating during
    night wakings, 49
  loveys, helping to ease, 76
  newborns, frequency of, 10
  short sleep cycles
    leading to, 47
noise factors, 5, 7, 11, 16, 70

O

overheating, 6, 14, 18

P

pacifiers, 11, 76, 77
play dates, avoiding during
  sleep training, 36
props. See sleep props

R

Rock 'N Play, 9
routines
  bedtime routines, 22, 26, 48
  books recommended for
    bedtime routine, 107
  laying baby down awake
    as last step of bedtime
    routine, 48–49
  naptime routine,
    importance of, 86
  for newborns, 10
  predictability as decreasing
    anxiety, 21

routines *(continued)*
restful activities as best for bedtime routines, 19
time changes, dealing with, 97

S

schedules
age-appropriate nap chart, 86
changing schedules, adapting to, 93
daylight saving time, taking into account, 97
internal clock readjustment, 95, 96
setting of schedules, 85
for six-month-olds, 22
traveling, maintaining schedule during, 101–2
weaning schedule, 82
security objects. *See* loveys
separation anxiety, 31, 35
setbacks, 99–103
siblings and sleep training, 41
skills, practice of, 31, 34, 35, 100
sleep journals, 5
sleep positioners and wedges, avoiding, 14
sleep props, 30, 55, 75–78
sleep sacks, 6, 91

sleep training chart, 32, 33
stroller walks, 7, 8, 10–11, 88
stuffed animals, 77
Sudden Infant Death Syndrome (SIDS)
car seats, sleeping in, 89
cribs as safest sleeping places, 9
loveys as risk factors, 76
overheating as a risk factor, 18
pacifiers as reducing risk of, 11
product claims, 14
room sharing as reducing risk of, 15
swaddling, 6, 7, 11
swings, 9, 88

T

teething, 103
travel, 36, 101–2

V

vaccinations, 102

W

wake-up time, adjusting, 96
weaning, 42, 80, 82, 83
white noise, 7, 11, 16

ACKNOWLEDGMENTS

I WANT TO THANK all of the sweet families that I have worked with over the years, who not only trusted me to work with the prized addition to their family—their baby—but who often welcomed me into their lives to share the joy and the tears of the sleep training journey. Sleep training is so much more than just helping a baby sleep. It's about helping a family unit that is often broken, in desperation, and at their wit's end; a family that is sleeping in separate beds, on the couch, even on the floor next to the baby just to survive; a family that is constantly anxious about bedtime, that forgot what a full night's rest, long shower, or date night even feels like. Who knew that a lack of sleep could have such a profound effect? If it weren't for all of you wonderful families who have shared your experiences with me, Sleep, Baby, Sleep® would have never come to fruition. I am grateful beyond words for you. Thank you for allowing me to help your family sleep better.

I also want to thank my daughters Brianna and Ava, who kept me up at all hours of the night, but led me to a deeper appreciation of the intricacy of sleep. It's because of them that I even know what sleep training is. Those sleepless nights were a real doozy, but I wouldn't have it any other way.

To all of my family and friends for supporting me through this writing process, cheering me on, and always having a glass of wine ready at the end of the week—I couldn't have completed this project without you!

ABOUT THE AUTHOR

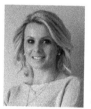

VIOLET GIANNONE is a registered nurse, pediatric sleep consultant, and founder of Sleep, Baby, Sleep®, a website dedicated to helping babies sleep. After struggling with getting her first baby to sleep, she faced immense sleep deprivation. Realizing that walking around like a zombie was no way to parent a baby, Violet developed a sleep training program that drew attention worldwide. Believing that "cry it out" is not the only way to help a baby sleep, Violet dedicated her time and research to developing a program that is gentle, yet effective. She is helping parents daily and all over the world through the VioletSleepBabySleep.com website. For a more tailored approach, she also offers personalized sleep plans and one-on-one consultations. Violet has been featured in, and is a pediatric sleep expert for, popular parenting websites such as Care.com, WhatToExpect.com, Moms Magazine.com, Macaroni Kid.com, Baby Chick.com, Tinyhood.com and more. When she is not helping babies sleep or busy running around with/after her two girls, Violet loves coffee, Mexican food, listening to loud music, dancing as if no one is watching, and always looking for opportunities to take the road less traveled.

CPSIA information can be obtained
at www.ICGtesting.com
Printed in the USA
BVHW06s0951280918
528441BV00008B/8/P

9 781641 521079